全国高职高专院校护理类专业核心教材

护理英语

（供护理、助产专业用）

主　编　胡晓莉　王筱楠
副主编　高秀桂　张媛媛
编　者　（以姓氏笔画为序）
　　　　王春霞（重庆三峡医药高等专科学校）
　　　　王筱楠（泰山护理职业学院）
　　　　关　庆（哈尔滨医科大学大庆校区）
　　　　李　娜（山东第一医科大学附属省立医院）
　　　　李晓宇（山东医学高等专科学校）
　　　　张媛媛（长沙卫生职业学院）
　　　　胡晓莉（山东医学高等专科学校）
　　　　徐　娟（重庆医药高等专科学校）
　　　　高秀桂（济南护理职业学院）
　　　　梁园荔（泰山护理职业学院）

U0232865

中国健康传媒集团
中国医药科技出版社

内 容 提 要

　　本教材为"全国高职高专院校护理类专业核心教材"之一，全书共九个单元，每单元主要包括阅读、听说、写作。其中每单元的听说部分由三个活动构成，每个活动按照护理程序由浅入深进行讲解。教材中的沟通技巧围绕单元主题，配合单元活动，把基本英语词汇和护理专业相结合使教材内容得到升华。教材的单元编排注重系统性、知识性与实用性。主要内容涉及收治新患者、用药护理、预防交叉感染；帮助患者准备检查、照护手术患者、出院护理、康复训练指导、提供社区照护和临终关怀等。本教材为书网融合教材，配套有数字教材、PPT 课件、微课、题库等数字化教学资源，使数字资源更多样化、立体化。

　　本教材可供全国高职高专院校护理、助产专业师生使用，也可作为护理行业职工培训、职业院校继续教育教材。

图书在版编目（CIP）数据

护理英语/胡晓莉，王筱楠主编．—北京：中国医药科技出版社，2022.2

全国高职高专院校护理类专业核心教材

ISBN 978 – 7 – 5214 – 2919 – 0

Ⅰ．①护…　Ⅱ．①胡…　②王…　Ⅲ．①护理学 – 英语 – 高等职业教育 – 教材　Ⅳ．①R47

中国版本图书馆 CIP 数据核字（2021）第 260371 号

美术编辑　陈君杞

版式设计　友全图文

出版　**中国健康传媒集团** | 中国医药科技出版社

地址　北京市海淀区文慧园北路甲 22 号

邮编　100082

电话　发行：010 – 62227427　邮购：010 – 62236938

网址　www.cmstp.com

规格　889mm × 1194mm $^{1}/_{16}$

印张　12

字数　351 千字

版次　2022 年 2 月第 1 版

印次　2022 年 2 月第 1 次印刷

印刷　三河市万龙印装有限公司

经销　全国各地新华书店

书号　ISBN 978 – 7 – 5214 – 2919 – 0

定价　**48.00** 元

获取新书信息、投稿、为图书纠错，请扫码联系我们。

出版说明

为了贯彻党的十九大精神，落实国务院《国家职业教育改革实施方案》文件精神，将"落实立德树人根本任务，发展素质教育"的战略部署要求贯穿教材编写全过程，充分体现教材育人功能，深入推动教学教材改革，中国医药科技出版社在院校调研的基础上，于2020年启动"全国高职高专院校护理类、药学类专业核心教材"的编写工作。在教育部、国家药品监督管理局的领导和指导下，在本套教材建设指导委员会和评审委员会等专家的指导和顶层设计下，根据教育部《职业教育专业目录（2021年）》要求，中国医药科技出版社组织全国高职高专院校及其附属机构历时1年精心编撰，现该套教材即将付梓出版。

本套教材包括护理类专业教材共计32门，主要供全国高职高专院校护理、助产专业教学使用；药学类专业教材33门，主要供药学类、中药学类、药品与医疗器械类专业师生教学使用。其中，为适应教学改革需要，部分教材建设为活页式教材。本套教材定位清晰、特色鲜明，主要体现在以下几个方面。

1. 体现职业核心能力培养，落实立德树人

教材应将价值塑造、知识传授和能力培养三者融为一体，融入思想道德教育、文化知识教育、社会实践教育，落实思想政治工作贯穿教育教学全过程。通过优化模块，精选内容，着力培养学生职业核心能力，同时融入企业忠诚度、责任心、执行力、积极适应、主动学习、创新能力、沟通交流、团队合作能力等方面的理念，培养具有职业核心能力的高素质技能型人才。

2. 体现高职教育核心特点，明确教材定位

坚持"以就业为导向，以全面素质为基础，以能力为本位"的现代职业教育教学改革方向，体现高职教育的核心特点，根据《高等职业学校专业教学标准》要求，培养满足岗位需求、教学需求和社会需求的高素质技术技能型人才，同时做到有序衔接中职、高职、高职本科，对接产业体系，服务产业基础高级化、产业链现代化。

3. 体现核心课程核心内容，突出必需够用

教材编写应能促进职业教育教学的科学化、标准化、规范化，以满足经济社会发展、产业升级对职业人才培养的需求，做到科学规划教材标准体系、准确定位教材核心内容，精炼基础理论知识，内容适度；突出技术应用能力，体现岗位需求；紧密结合各类职业资格认证要求。

4.体现数字资源核心价值，丰富教学资源

提倡校企"双元"合作开发教材，积极吸纳企业、行业人员加入编写团队，引入一些岗位微课或者视频，实现岗位情景再现；提升知识性内容数字资源的含金量，激发学生学习兴趣。免费配套的"医药大学堂"数字平台，可展现数字教材、教学课件、视频、动画及习题库等丰富多样、立体化的教学资源，帮助老师提升教学手段，促进师生互动，满足教学管理需要，为提高教育教学水平和质量提供支撑。

编写出版本套高质量教材，得到了全国知名专家的精心指导和各有关院校领导与编者的大力支持，在此一并表示衷心感谢。出版发行本套教材，希望得到广大师生的欢迎，对促进我国高等职业教育护理类和药学类相关专业教学改革和人才培养做出积极贡献。希望广大师生在教学中积极使用本套教材并提出宝贵意见，以便修订完善，共同打造精品教材。

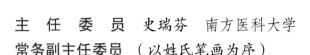

贾　强　山东药品食品职业学院

高璀乡　江苏医药职业学院

葛淑兰　山东医学高等专科学校

韩忠培　浙江药科职业大学

覃晓龙　遵义医药高等专科学校

委　　　员（以姓氏笔画为序）

王庭之　江苏医药职业学院

兰作平　重庆医药高等专科学校

司　毅　山东医学高等专科学校

朱扶蓉　福建卫生职业技术学院

刘　亮　遵义医药高等专科学校

刘林凤　山西药科职业学院

李　明　济南护理职业学院

李　媛　江苏食品药品职业技术学院

孙　萍　重庆三峡医药高等专科学校

何　雄　浙江药科职业大学

何文胜　福建生物工程职业技术学院

沈　伟　山东中医药高等专科学校

沈必成　楚雄医药高等专科学校

张　虹　长春医学高等专科学校

张奎升　山东药品食品职业学院

张钱友　长沙卫生职业学院

张雷红　广东食品药品职业学院

陈　亚　邢台医学高等专科学校

陈　刚　赣南卫生健康职业学院

罗　翀　湖南食品药品职业学院

郝晶晶　北京卫生职业学院

胡莉娟　杨凌职业技术学院

徐贤淑　辽宁医药职业学院

高立霞　山东医药技师学院

康　伟　天津生物工程职业技术学院

傅学红　益阳医学高等专科学校

数字化教材编委会

主　编　胡晓莉　王筱楠

副主编　高秀桂　张媛媛

编　者　（以姓氏笔画为序）

王春霞（重庆三峡医药高等专科学校）

王筱楠（泰山护理职业学院）

关　庆（哈尔滨医科大学大庆校区）

李　娜（山东第一医科大学附属省立医院）

李晓宇（山东医学高等专科学校）

张媛媛（长沙卫生职业学院）

胡晓莉（山东医学高等专科学校）

徐　娟（重庆医药高等专科学校）

高秀桂（济南护理职业学院）

梁园荔（泰山护理职业学院）

前　言

　　《护理英语》为"全国高职高专院校护理类专业核心教材"之一，根据高职院校人才培养目标和主要就业方向及护理职业能力要求，按照本套教材编写指导思想和原则要求，结合《高等职业教育英语课程教学基本要求》和护理英语课程教学大纲，尝试对接国际领域的权威职业英语技能认证考试（OET：Occupational English Test for Nursing）考核标准，由全国 7 所院校和 1 所三级甲等医院从事教学和生产一线的教师、行业专家悉心编写而成。旨在培养学生在真实工作场景下运用专业英语的技能，从而提高学生的职业胜任力，为学生未来职业生涯和职业能力的可持续发展奠定坚实的基础，迎合全球经济一体化以及中国"一带一路"国家战略的成功实施带来的国际医疗卫生事业发展的新趋势、新契机和新挑战。适用于全国高职高专院校护理类各专业教学。

　　本教材为山东省教育科学"十三五"规划课题"基于职业资格标准的高职英语课程改革研究（2020WGYB012）"系列成果之一。内容设置围绕"以了解和满足人的需求为出发点"的全生命周期护理观，按照 OET 护理测试相关工作领域和临床护理工作岗位过程分为"三个活动模块"，即"门诊护理""住院护理"和"社区家庭护理"。三者呈现递进关系，帮助护生完成一个人从疾病到健康的全过程护理，提炼出 9 个典型工作任务，分别包括收治新患者、用药护理、预防交叉感染、帮助患者准备检查、照护手术患者、出院护理、康复训练指导、提供社区照护和临终关怀。在选材中融入了《国家护士执业资格考试大纲》（2020 版）的部分内容，并与澳大利亚开发的 OET 考试中针对护理专业的内容和形式进行对接，选取与护理专业职场环境下具有实用价值的英文素材，突出医学特色和实用性，强调语言学习的最终目标是用语言表达、交流思想和信息。

　　本教材为"教学做一体化"教材。全书共 9 个单元，每个单元设计为 4 学时，可以根据不同专业需要选择合适的内容，各单元的具体内容如下。

　　单元热身（Warm - up exercises）：图文配对，以实际工作任务引入单元主题相关、最具代表性的知识点。

　　阅读部分（Reading）：课文主要选自与单元主题相关的国内外英文刊物。注释（Notes）针对文章中出现的专业问题和特别的语言点提供了必要的解释。课后习题（After - reading Exercise）包括配对练习、填空和简答练习。

　　听说部分（Listening & Speaking）：分为 3 个活动，每个活动均围绕单元主题相关的职场情境，呈递进逻辑关系。

　　活动 1~3（Activity 1~3）：每个活动包括 4~5 个任务，前几个任务都设有注释（Notes），解释专业难点和语言点。最后一个任务是口语，根据听力内容设计，帮助学生将听力中的专业语言点内化为自己的语言表达能力。

　　沟通技巧（Communication Tips）：每个活动最后都设置了专业沟通技巧。帮助学生提升沟通能力，建立平等良好的治疗性护患关系。

　　写作部分（Writing）：写作内容结合单元主题，完成实践工作场景中的涉及各种题材，如用药记录、出院记录、热点讨论等。

　　谚语俗语（Proverbs and Sayings）：护理专业相关谚语俗语，有助于了解医学相关文化，同时提高学生的职业荣誉感。

　　本教材主要供全国高职高专院校护理类、助产类专业师生使用，也可作为医学护理行业职工培训、职业院校继续教育课程使用。本教材由胡晓莉和王筱楠担任主编。胡晓莉负责拟定本书的编写提纲、编写体例、编写样章。王筱楠负责数字化资源样例。高秀桂、张媛媛、李晓宇和梁园荔老师负责全书统稿、数字化资源和微课审核。每位老师都参与了教材审稿的工作。具体编写分工如下：单元 1 由王筱楠编写；单元 2 由胡晓莉编写；单元 3 由关庆编写；单元 4 由王春霞编写；单元 5 由李晓宇和李娜编写；单元 6 由梁园荔编写；单元 7 由张媛媛编写；单元 8 由徐娟编写；单元 9 由高秀桂编写；各位老师同时还承担了相应单元的数字化资源编写。全体编写团队老师牺牲大量个人时间，为本书的编写付出辛勤的劳动和心血，在此表示衷心的感谢。

　　本教材在编写过程中得到了编写团队所在单位的领导、老师和技术人员的热情支持和帮助，在此一并表示衷心的感谢。由于编者水平有限，疏漏之处在所难免，恳请广大读者及各方面的专家、学者提出宝贵意见，以便进一步修改完善。

编　者

2021 年 12 月

目 录

Unit 1　Admitting Patients

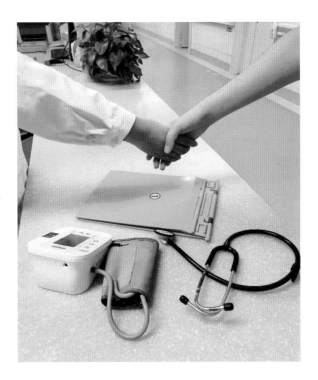

Learning Objectives

Reading part：

Be able to identify the details of admission procedure.

Listening and Speaking part：

1. Be able to welcome a patient on admission.

2. Be able to perform the admission procedure.

3. Be able to introduce the ward to the patients.

4. Be able to collect correct information by using and admission form.

5. Be able to use effective communication strategies to improve the nurse – patient relationship.

Writing part：

Be able to write an admission report with appropriate medical English.

Warm – up Exercises

If you go to see a doctor, you'd better bring the following things. Match the pictures with these items.

| ID card Outpatient medical record Medical insurance card |

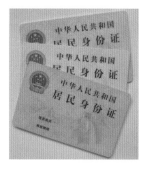

A _____

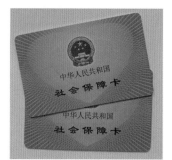

B _____

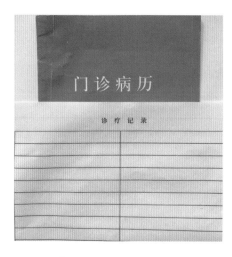

C _____

Reading

阅读译文

Hospital Admission Procedure

Usually a patient is received in hospital either in general outpatient department (OPD) or in Emergency. The details of a nurse's responsibility while the patient is admitted to hospital are being described below.

Welcoming a patient on admission

Receive the patient into the system in such a manner that he/she feels welcome and secure while comfort, safety, biopsychosocial, cultural, financial and spiritual needs are addressed; and obtain the key information identified to process the patient admission. If the patient is in walking condition, allow him to sit on a stool or chair. If the patient is in stretcher, shift him to an examining bed. If the patient is carried by attendants or relatives by physically lifting with arms support, allow the patient to sit or lie down on a bed depending upon the condition.

Filling in the admission form

Before the patient is taken to his ward, admitting procedures are performed. The patient's personal data is recorded and entered into the hospital's computer system.

There may be several forms to fill out. One form may be a detailed medical and medication history. This history will include past hospitalizations and surgeries. Having this information readily available will make the process move faster, and can allow a family member or friend who is accompanying the patient to help fill out the forms more easily.

Another form is called a living will and clearly tells which specific resuscitation efforts the person does or does not want to have performed on them in order to save or extend their life.

Taking the patients to the ward

Once all the admitting information has been completed, the next step is usually taking the patient to the ward. The nurse taking care of the patient will orient the person to the ward. This means that they will explain how to adjust bed height, how to use the nurse call button, how to use the bedside telephone and television and show where the bathroom is located.

The nurse will review the doctor's orders, such as what tests have been scheduled, whether or not they can get out of bed for the bathroom or to walk around the ward, what medications they will be getting, and whether or not there are restrictions on what they can eat.

(381 words)

Notes

1. Welcoming a patient on admission 欢迎患者入院

本句中"admission"意为"入院"。"admission"为名词, 动词为"admit"医学英语中常用的表达为"be admitted to", 意为"被收治入院"。

e. g. He was admitted to the hospital last week. 他上周被收治入院。

Many patients are trapped in a revolving door of admission, discharge, and readmission. 许多患者陷入入院、出院、再入院的怪圈里。

2. Receive the patient into the system in such a manner that he/she feels welcome and secure while comfort, safety, biopsychosocial, cultural, financial and spiritual needs are addressed.

在满足舒适、安全、生物心理社会、文化、经济和精神需求的同时, 让患者以一种让他/她感到受欢迎和安全的方式收治入院。

本句重点强调在同患者交流的过程中, 需要考虑患者的身份、文化背景, 尊重其心理要求, 以恰当有效的方式与其交谈, 建立轻松愉悦的交流氛围。

3. The nurse taking care of the patient will orient the person to the ward.

负责患者的护士会给患者介绍病房的情况。

本句中"orient"意为"使熟悉, 帮助适应"。

e. g. The first days of school are meant to orient the freshmen to campus life.

开学头几天用来让新学生熟悉校园生活。

4. If the patient is in stretcher, shift him to an examining bed.

如果患者是平车运送入院, 把他转移到检查床上。

本句中"shift… to"意为"转到"。

e. g. He shifted the load from his left shoulder to his right.

他把扛的东西从左肩换到右肩。

After – reading Exercises

Task 1   Match the words with their proper meanings.

1. outpatient department	a. 医嘱
2. call button	b. 抢救，复苏
3. biopsychosocial	c. 用药史
4. personal data	d. 平车，担架
5. living will	e. 病房
6. ward	f. 生前遗嘱
7. stretcher	g. 个人信息
8. medication history	h. 生物心理社会的
9. resuscitation	i. 呼叫器
10. doctor's orders	j. 门诊

Task 2   Complete the following sentences with a word or short phrase from the text.

1. Nurses should make the patient feel welcome and _____ when they are admitted into hospital.

2. If the patient can walk by himself, allow him to _____ a stool or chair.

3. Admitting procedures should _____, before the patient is taken to the ward.

4. The detailed medical and medication will include _____ .

5. The nurse will tell the patient how to adjust bed height and show where the bathroom _____ .

Task 3   In pairs, discuss the following questions.

1. What kind of forms should the nurse fill in when admitting the patients?

_____

_____

_____

2. Do you know the communication manners with patients when they are on admission? What are they?

_____

_____

_____

_____

Listening and Speaking

Activity 1   Welcoming a Patient on Admission

Task 1   The following abbreviations and terms are commonly used on admission forms. Work in pairs, match 1 ~ 10 with a ~ j.

1. I. D. No.	a. Pulse
2. P	b. Blood Pressure
3. BP	c. Respiratory Rate
4. RR	d. Temperature
5. T	e. Identification Number
6. Family History	f. The total sum of a patient's health status prior to the presenting problem
7. Allergic History	g. Allergic reactions happened in the past
8. Past Medical History	h. Health information about disorders from which the direct blood relatives of the patient have suffered
9. Chief Complaints	i. A group of the important medical signs that indicate the status of the body's vital (life – sustaining) functions
10. Vital Signs	j. A concise statement of the symptoms that caused a patient to seek medical care

Notes

At the time of admission, the nurses collected the data of the patients according to the admission form. Nurses will make a nursing plan according to valuation of the health status of patients, the physical condition, psychological needs and health problems of patients.

在患者入院时，护士根据入院表格收集患者的个人信息。护士根据患者的健康状况、身体状况、心理需求和健康问题的评估，制定护理计划。

Task 2   In pairs, discuss the registration card below and point out what the letters 'A – F' stand for.

Registration card

A *Paul*

B *Male*

C *5 th, May, 1961*

D   *No. 45 Shandong Road, Jiangzhou*

E *799 – 01160*

F *penicillin*

Notes

1. "Registration card" 是指挂号单，患者在初次就诊挂号时需要填写的。

2. 填写出生日期，英语中有几种填写方式。可以写成：5th，May，1961 或者 05/05/1961。

Task 3 Listen to a conversation between a nurse and a patient, then fill into the blanks.

听力 1.1

1. What seems to be _____ you?

2. Please pay ten yuan for the _____ .

3. Please take the elevator to the _____ and then turn right.

4. Go along the _____ until you see the sign on your left.

5. OK, don't worry. I will make an _____ for you.

Notes

1. 英语口语询问病情还可以这样表达：

What's the matter with you?

What's your trouble?

What's wrong with you?

What's your problem?

2. registration 意为"挂号"。

Task 4 Listen and complete. In pairs, talk about some information about Leo. Then fill the blanks.

| Leo's chief complaint：（1）_____ |
| （2）_____ |
| （3）_____ |
| （4）_____ |

听力 1.1

| Leo has been ill since（5）_____ . |

| Leo has been here（6）_____ and this is his（7）_____ visit here. |

| Leo should register with（8）_____ . |

Notes

1. "complaint" 意为"主诉"。除此之外还有"投诉""抱怨"之意。

e. g. Once you receive a client complaint, deal with it as fast as you can.

一旦接到客户投诉，要尽快处理。

2. "soreness" 意为"疼痛"。其形容词为"sore"，一般指"肌肉疼痛"。

e. g. I have a sore throat. 我喉咙疼痛。

3. "medical department" 意为"内科"。医院里其他科室表达如：surgical department（外科），pediatrics department（小儿科），dental department（牙科）等。

4. "register with" 意为"挂（某科）的号"。

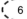

Task 5   **Work in groups, make a dialogue between a nurse and a patient with the following information. Swap roles and practice again.**

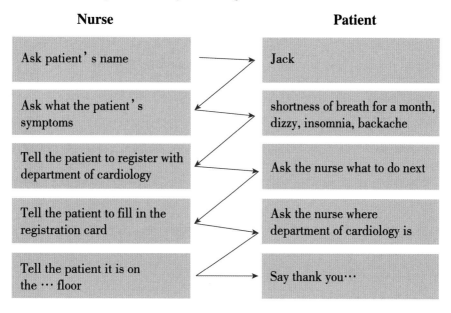

Communication Tips:

When welcoming patients on admission, you meet different people everyday. After someone greets you, it is important to respond appropriately. Here are some common responses to greet.

Formal	Informal
I am doing great.	Not too bad. Pretty good.
How are you keeping?	How are you doing?
It is so nice to see you.	Nice to see you.
It has been a long time since we met last time.	Long time no see.

Listening and Speaking

Activity 2   Going through the Admission Procedure

Task 1   **Match the abbreviations (1 ~ 5) with expressions (a ~ e).**

1. ID bracelet	a. bed number
2. DOB	b. date of birth
3. ADM	c. admission date
4. Dr.	d. doctor
5. Bed. No.	e. identity bracelet

✂ Notes

在医院中，住院的患者手上戴着腕带，以便于能够让医生核对患者身份，而部分识别腕带上便于移动设备扫码，这个二维码能够记录患者的基本信息，其中包括姓名、年龄、血型、身份证号等，而且还包括一些病史等医疗信息，可以帮助医生全面性的了解患者，从而进行更准确的诊断和治疗。

Task 2 Listen to the conversation and complete the following extracts.

听力 1.2

Ann：Good morning, Mr. Paul. My name is Ann and I will be one of the nurses

(1) _____ you here.

Mr. Paul：Nice to meet you, Ann. Would you please tell me where I should go for the

(2) _____ ?

Ann：Here. Would you mind showing me your outpatient (3) _____ .

Mr. Paul：Here you are.

Ann：Before your admission, I'd like to ask you some questions.

Mr. Paul：OK. What would you like to know?

Ann：Would you please tell me your (4) _____ and (5) _____ ?

Mr. Paul：It's Chris Paul and I was born on (6) _____ .

✂ Notes

"Would you please …" 用于请求别人帮忙，表示"你愿意……吗"？是一种委婉的表达方式。类似的句型还有"Would you like to …"在护患交流过程中，护士一定注意语言修养，注意语言礼貌性，多用安慰语、鼓励话。同时还要注意眼神的交流和面部表情变化。

Task 3 Listen to the conversation again and answer the following questions.

听力 1.2

(1) Where does Mr. Paul live?

_____

_____

(2) Why did Mr. Paul have an operation two years ago?

_____

_____

(3) What kind of medicine is he allergic to?

_____

_____

(4) Why does the nurse take his vital signs?

_____

_____

✂ Notes

1. "operation" 手术。动词为"operate"，例如"operate on sb"是"给某人做手术"。

e. g. We will have to operate on his eyes. 我们得给他的眼睛做手术。

2. "be allergic to" 对……过敏。

e. g. The boy is allergic to seafood. 男孩对海鲜过敏。

Task 4   Listen again. Fill in the data of vital signs of Mr. Paul.

听力 1.2

BP	1.
P	2.
T	3.
RR	4.

Notes

1. "bradycardia" 意为 "心动过缓"。"brady –" 前缀意为 "慢的"。前缀在单词中位于词根前面的部分，常改变词义。

e. g. bradydiastole 心舒张期延长

2. "RR" 为 "Respiratory rate" 的缩写，译为 "呼吸频率"。

Task 5   In pairs, make a dialogue. Use Task 2 as a guide. Use the following prompts to help you. Swap roles and practice again.

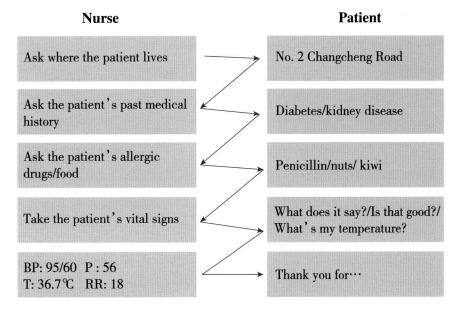

Communication Tips：

Authentic Oral Expression in Hospital Admission

The relationship between nurses and patients is becoming more and more important, while the communication between them takes a critical place in clinical nursing work.

1. A kind smile, warm words and thoughtful introduction, combined with appropriate body language will make the patients feel valued like going home.

2. Approachable tone and intonation are used to provide supportive language to show the maximum understanding of patients. Patients can naturally express their thoughts and feelings in a relaxed atmosphere of conversation.

3. It is important for the nurse to be good at listening in communicating with patients, for half of the effect of the conversation depends on listening. Sit down, listen patiently, and respond to what the patient said.

Listening and Speaking

Activity 3   Taking Patients to the Ward

Task 1   Look at the pictures and tell your partner what the picture is mainly about.

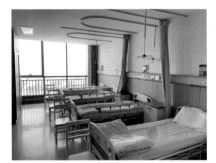
A _____

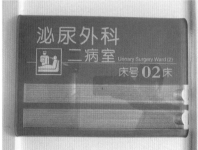
B _____

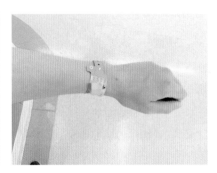
C _____

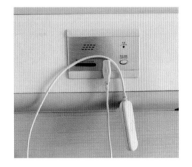
D _____

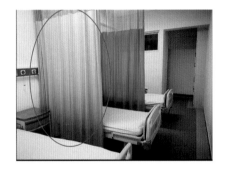
E _____

✖ Notes

Ward nurses introduce hospitalization rules to patients and help them get familiar with the environment. Good admission introduction can fully mobilize the subjective activity of patients and make them in the best state of receiving treatment and nursing during the whole hospitalization period, so as to recover as soon as possible.

病房护士向患者介绍住院期间的规定，协助患者熟悉环境。良好的入院介绍可以充分调动患者的主观能动性，使其在住院期间保持治疗和护理的最佳状态，以利于早日康复。

Task 2   Listen to the conversation and complete the following extracts.

听力 1.3

1. Doctor Li asked Lucy to take an _____ for Mr. Smith.

2. Mr. Smith needs to have a _____ in the chest radiography room.

3. The chest radiography room is on the _____ floor.

4. Mr. Smith is diagnosed with _____ disease.

✂ **Notes**

1. be responsible for 意为 "为……负责"。

    e. g.　I would be responsible for my actions if I saw him.

    如果我看到他，我会为我的行为负责。

2. ward rounds：意为 "查房"。

    e. g.　make ward rounds 查房

🎧 **Task 3**　**Listen to the conversation and decide the following sentences are true or false. Write "T" for true or "F" for false.**

听力 1.3

☐（1）You can take off your wrist bracelet in the ward.

☐（2）There is a single room in the ward.

☐（3）At 3 o'clock in the afternoon, Mr. Smith needs to have a chest X – ray.

☐（4）The ward rounds and treatment start at 9 am.

☐（5）Mr. Smith has a heart problem for many years.

✂ **Notes**

ECG examination：意为 "心电图检查"。ECG 是 electrocardiogram 的缩写形式。一般的医学词汇比较长，但是很多词汇是由词根和词缀组成。在 "electrocardiogram" 中，cardio 是词根，意思是 "心脏的"，gram 是后缀，意思是 "记录，写或画出来的东西"。例如：cardialgia 心痛；myogram 肌动图。

🎧 **Task 4**　**Listen to the conversation and answer the following questions.**

听力 1.4

（1）What's Mr. Smith's bed number?

_____

_____

_____

（2）Why didn't Mr. Smith sleep well last night?

_____

_____

_____

（3）How is Mr. Smith's appetite? And why should he eat more vegetables and fruit?

_____

_____

_____

（4）What does Mr. Smith feel all the time? What treatments will the nurse take?

_____

_____

_____

✂ **Notes**

nursing ward rounds：护理查房

随着患者对医疗、护理乃至后勤服务等方面需求的不断提高，护士的角色也由过去的单一化逐渐向多型化转变。每日护理查房对妥善地处理好护患关系，促进患者的康复、保证护理工作的质量以及减少医疗纠纷的发生产生积极的效果。护士查房内容一般包括患者的饮食、睡眠、大小便等日常起居方面，叮嘱患者按时服药，健康饮食等。

Task 5 In pairs, make a dialogue. Use the following information to help you. Swap roles and practice again.

Suppose that you are a ward nurse in Neurology department. A patient is admitted in this department. Introduce the ward, ward rounds, physical condition and treatment options to the patient. Tell the patient dos and donts when in the ward.

When a nurse introduces the ward, ward rounds, and treatment options to the patient, she often says：	There is a curtain, you can pull it around the bed… You can push the button if … The visiting hours are from… to … The ward rounds and treatment start at… The patient need take an ECG examination / have a chest X – ray…
When a nurse tells the patient dos and donts in the ward, she often says：	You'd better eat some vegetables /fruit. You have to rest in bed/have a rest. You'd better not stay up late.

Communication Tips：

Nurses should pay attention to the ways of communication when introducing the ward to the patients.

1. When tell the patients some dos and donts, daily language should be used.

2. The popularization of medical terms is easy for patients to remember.

3. For the patients with high acceptance ability and high education level, make them know their own condition, diagnosis, treatment. Otherwise, nurses should patiently guide the diet, introduce the doctor in charge.

To high education and acceptance ability patients：

You are diagnosed as coronary heart disease.

The test findings of your kidney functions have just got normal.

This medicine is used for preventing infection.

To low education and acceptance ability patients：

You should have light food, a lot of vegetables and fruits.

Too much salt will hurt your kidney, so you need to be careful about having salt.

Doctor Smith will be in charge of you.

Writing

Finish a patient report on his admission information based on the following table.

Patient admission form	
Patient name：John Smith Admission date：September 7th Bed No. ：65	Initial complains：difficulty breathing, vomit once every another hour, abdominal pain, diarrhea
Age ：18	Gender：male
Signs & symptoms：T 40°C, P 94/min, RR 20/min, BP 123/80mmHg	
Possible problems：risk of dehydration	
Nursing instructions：bed rest for 2 days, drink much fluid and daily fluid intake of 2500ml	

Proverbs and Sayings

❖ To rescue the wounded, time is life. To save a wounded person and reduce his pain is the greatest happiness of our medical workers.

对抢救伤员来说，时间就是生命，能抢救一个伤员，为伤员减少一份痛苦，就是我们医务工作者最大的快乐。

❖ In a hospital, there is one person who is very responsible, and everyone will benefit, and one person who is not responsible, and everyone may get harm.

一个医院里，有一个人很负责任，大家都会得到好处，有一个人不负责任，大家都有可能得到坏处。

❖ I will be pure all my life, faithful to my duties, and do my best to raise the standard of care; do not take or use harmful drugs for harm; keep the patient's household chores and secrets carefully, and assist the doctor in his treatment and in his welfare.

终身纯洁，忠贞职守，尽力提高护理之标准；勿为有损之事，勿取服或故用有害之药；慎守患者家务及秘密，竭诚协助医生之诊治，勿谋病者之福利。

书网融合……

听力材料1.1

听力材料1.2

听力材料1.3

听力材料1.4

Unit 2　Administering Medications

PPT

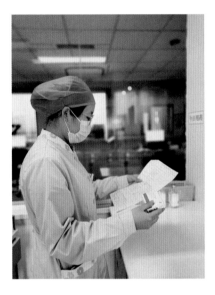

Reading part:

Be able to identify the details of safe medication administration.

Listening and Speaking part:

1. Be able to identify and recognize specific information on medical prescriptions.

2. Be able to correctly explain prescriptions to other healthcare providers, using effective communication strategies within a multidisciplinary team.

3. Be able to apply the five rights of medication administration when two nurses do a medication check.

4. Be able to communicate with another nurse during medication check procedures, using communication tips for working as part of a team.

5. Be able to identify and recognize specific information about safe medication administration.

6. Be able to correctly explain medication usage according to medical record, using effective communication strategies, and building a therapeutic relationship.

Writing part:

Be able to write a medication administration record which is clinical and factual, using appropriate medical terminology, accurate grammar and punctuation.

Warm – up Exercises

Nancy is a nurse who is responsible for preparing medication for the patients. Can you help her to label the different types of medication and explain the correct administration route?

Liquid	Tablet	Capsule	Topical medicine	
Suppository	Drop	Inhaler	Injection	Patch

A

B

C

D

E

F

G

H

I

Reading

阅读译文

Medication Safety: Go beyond the Basics

For any nurse working in a direct care setting, preparing medications and administering them to patients is part of the daily routine. Mistakes can happen at any point in the process. Administration errors are one of the most serious and most common mistakes made by nurses. The result may lengthen a hospital stay, increase costs, or have life and death implications for the patient. So, what can you do to administer medications safely?

Start with the basics

◇ Verify any medication order and make sure it's complete. The order should include the drug name, dosage, frequency, and route of administration. If any element is missing, check with the practitioner.

◇ Check the patient's medical record for an allergy or contraindication to the prescribed medication.

◇ Prepare medications for one patient at a time.

◇ Educate patients about their medications. Encourage them to speak up if something seems amiss.

Minimize distractions and interruptions

◇ Know that interruptions and distractions have a marked effect on your performance, causing a lack of attention, forgetfulness, and errors.

◇ Make sure you have all the required supplies and documents available before beginning preparation or administration activities.

Implement these additional safety measures

◇ Be especially alert during high – risk situations, such as when you are stressed, tired, or angry, or when supervising inexperienced personnel.

◇ Be familiar with all appropriate antidotes, reversal agents, and rescue agents. Know where they are stored on your unit and how to administer them in an emergency situation.

◇ Measure and document a patient's weight in metric units (grams and kilograms) ONLY to allow for accurate dosage calculations. Also, weigh the patient as soon as possible on admission and don't rely on stated, estimated, or historical weights.

◇ For patients receiving IV opioid medication, frequently monitor respiratory rate, sedation level, and oxygen saturation level or exhaled carbon dioxide to decrease the risk of adverse reactions associated with IV opioid use.

◇ Administer high – alert intravenous medication infusions via a programmable infusion device utilizing dose error reduction software.

◇ Reconcile the patient's medications at each care transition and when a new medication is ordered to reduce the risk for medication errors, including omissions, duplications, dosing errors, and drug interactions.

◇ Educate and provide written instructions to the patient and family (or caregiver) regarding prescribed medications for use when at home and verify their understanding prior to discharge.

(398 words)

✂ Notes

1. Preparing medications and administering them to patients is the part of the daily routine. 准备药物并给患者用药是日常工作的一部分。

本句中"administer"应翻译为"（医生，护士，药剂师等）派发（药物）"。所以请注意医务人员进行"发药"这个专业任务，应该表达为"administer medicine"，而"give medicine"则强调医务人员将药物给予患者服用或使用的动作。

e. g. The physician prescribes the drug and the nurse administers it.

医生负责开处方药而护士负责发药。

2. The order should include the drug name, dosage, frequency and route of administration. 医嘱应包括药名、剂量、给药频率和给药途径。

本句中"order"应翻译为"医嘱"而不是"命令"。医嘱的主要内容包括"患者"和"药物"信息。护理人员在执行医嘱时需要严格遵守查对制度，在我国，护理人员通常使用"三查七对"药物核对制度。三查七对通常翻译为"three inspections and seven verifications"，三查包括"操作前查、操作中查和操作后查"即"inspect before administering medicine; inspect during administering medicine; inspect after administering medicine"，七对包括核对"床号、姓名、药名、浓度、剂量、方法和时间"即 verify "bed number; patient's name; drug name; drug saturation; drug dosage; route and time"。

3. Be familiar with all appropriate antidotes, reversal agents, and rescue agents.

熟悉所有正确的解毒药、逆转药和抢救药。

"be familiar with"熟悉，熟知

e. g. Nurses must be familiar with acute kidney injury guidelines.

护士必须熟悉急性肾损伤指南。

"antidotes"是指"解毒药"，英文解释是"Antidoteis a chemical substance that stops or controls the effect of a poison."中文解释是"它是一种化学物质，可以停止或控制毒药的作用。"例如"Acetylcysteine for acetaminophen poisoning."，即"乙酰半胱氨酸用于对乙酰氨基酚中毒。"

"reversal agents"是指"逆转药"，英文解释是"Reversal agents are defined as any drug used to reverse the effects of anesthetics, narcotics or potentially toxic agents."中文解释是"逆转剂定义为用于逆转麻醉剂，麻醉毒品或潜在毒性剂作用的任何药物。"例如"Naloxone, reverses the effects of opioids."，即"纳洛酮，逆转阿片类药物的作用。"

"rescue agents"是指"抢救药"，英文解释是"Rescue agents are defined as medicine intended to relieve symptoms immediately."中文解释是"抢救药定义为可以立即缓解症状的药物。"例如"Epinephrine is used to stop severe allergic reactions (anaphylaxis)"，即"肾上腺素用于阻止严重的过敏反应（过敏）。"

4. Administer high - alert intravenous medication infusions via a programmable infusion device utilizing dose error reduction software.

在静脉注射高风险药物时，使用带有减少剂量误差软件的可编程输液装置。

"high - alert medication"是指"高危药物"，这些药物在使用过程中一旦用药错误是会极大增加患者受严重伤害的风险。即使这些错误在用药过程中可能并不常见，但是一旦出现差错，对患者造成的伤害是可以致命的。根据研究，常见的高危药物包括"insulin, opiates and narcotics, injectable potassium chloride (or phosphate) concentrate, intravenous anticoagulants (heparin), and sodium chloride solutions above 0.9%"，即"胰岛素，鸦片和麻醉剂，可注射的氯化钾（或磷酸盐）浓缩液，静脉内抗凝剂（肝素）和0.9%以上的氯化钠溶液"。

After – reading Exercises

Task 1   Match the words with their proper meanings.

1. Administration	a. 核实
2. Verify	b. 过敏
3. Dosage	c. 禁忌证
4. Route	d. 鸦片样物质
5. Allergy	e. 不良反应
6. Contraindication	f. 途径
7. Antidote	g. 解毒药
8. Opioid	h. 剂量
9. Adverse Reaction	i. 镇静
10. Sedation	j. 派发药物

Task 2   Complete the following sentences with a word or short phrase from the text.

1. When you verify the order, you should check the drug name, ＿＿＿＿＿＿, frequency, and route of administration.

2. Patients are not allowed to take medicine if they have an ＿＿＿＿＿＿ or contraindication to the prescribed medication.

3. Nurses are more likely to make medical errors if they prepare medications for more than ＿＿＿＿＿＿ patient at a time.

4. For a patient who takes the poisons, nurses must know where the ＿＿＿＿＿＿ are stored and how to administer them to him/her.

5. According to the passage, patients receiving IV opioid medication are more likely to suffer from ＿＿＿＿＿＿ distress because of the adverse reactions of IV opioid use.

Task 3   In pairs, discuss the following questions.

1. Do you think medication safety is important? Why?

＿＿

＿＿

2. Being a nurse, what are the responsibilities for administering medications?

＿＿

＿＿

＿＿

Listening and Speaking

Activity 1　Identifying Prescription

Task 1　The following abbreviations are commonly used on prescription charts. Work in pairs, match the terms and abbreviations (1 ~ 16) with expressions (a ~ p).

Route of Drug Administration	
1. IM	a. intravenous injection
2. IV	b. subcutaneous injection
3. SC	c. intradermal injection
4. ID	d. intramuscular injection
5. PO	e. by mouth
Timing and Frequency of an Order	
6. qd	f. three times a day
7. bid	g. four times a day
8. tid	h. twice a day
9. qid	i. every other day
10. qod	j. once a day
11. 6/24	k. every six hours
12. qh	l. every hour
13. hs	m. before meals
14. ac	n. after meals
15. pc	o. at bedtime
16. prn	p. as needed

✖ Notes

Abbreviations are commonly used in the medical world to save time and space whilst writing in the patients' medical records. It takes less time to say or write an abbreviated form of the full word than to spell out every single word. So, using abbreviations in your everyday speech makes communication easier and faster.

在医学领域中通常使用缩写来节省书写病历的时间和空间。说或写出完整单词的缩写形式所花的时间少于说出每个单词所花费的时间。因此，在日常讲话中使用缩写可以使交流变得更加轻松和快捷。

Task 2　In pairs, discuss the prescription below and point out what the letters 'A – I' stand for.

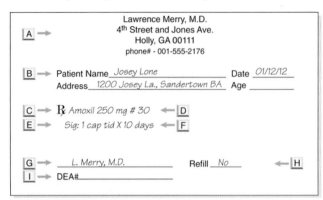

✎ Notes

1. A prescription, often abbreviated ℞ or Rx, is a health care program implemented by a physician or other qualified health care practitioner in the form of instructions that govern the plan of care for an individual patient. It normally includes three parts: doctor information, patient information, and drug information.

处方，通常缩写为℞或 Rx，是由医生或其他有资质的医疗保健从业人员制定的方案，用于指导患者的治疗。它通常包括三个部分：医生信息，患者信息和药物信息。

2. 'Sig' is short for the Latin 'Signa or Signaturaor', which means 'let it be labeled'.

"Sig"是拉丁文"Signa or Signatura"的缩写，是指"用法"，建议严格遵医嘱用药。

3. "refill"是指医生对于患者使用处方次数的授权，如果 refill 后面的次数是"1"，即患者在服用完药后，可带着处方到药房再拿同等剂量的药物 1 次而不需要找医生重新开医嘱。如果后面的次数写的是"No/None"，就表示患者在服用完药物后，需要到医生那里复查，不能再去药房取药了。

4. "DEA"是"Drug Enforcement Administration（美国禁毒署）"的缩写。如果医生开的处方药是管制药品，如毒麻药，医生需在签名旁注明美国禁毒署授权给他的 DEA 号。

Task 3　In pairs, read the prescription and write them out in words. Then listen and check your answer.

听力 2.1

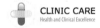

CLINIC CARE
Health and Clinical Excellence

Name: **Brian McCallister** Age:

℞

Amoxicillin 400 mg/5 ml

Sig 5 ml PO BID x 10 days

Dispense 100 mL

Refills: None

Brand name medically necessary

Signature

25, Imperial Drive, NY 21784

1. Brian McCallister needs to take ＿＿＿＿＿＿ of amoxicillin ＿＿＿＿＿＿ a day for ＿＿＿＿＿＿ days.

2. The amoxicillin will be taken by ＿＿＿＿＿＿ .

3. The doctor dispense ＿＿＿＿＿＿ of amoxicillin to Brian McCallister this time. Once the patient takes all the drugs, he needs to go back to the ＿＿＿＿＿＿ rather than a pharmacy.

4. The doctor will prescribe the drug with a ＿＿＿＿＿＿ name and prohibit the substitution of a generi-cally equivalent drug.

✎ Notes

1. "amoxicillin" 是指药物"阿莫西林", 是一种最常用的半合成青霉素类广谱 β – 内酰胺类抗生素。

2. "dispense" 是指 "give or apply (medications)", 即发药。

3. "Brand name" 是指药品的"商品名", 是由不同药品生产厂商对于自己制剂产品所起的名字, 具有专用权。"generic name" 是指药品的"化学名"或"通用名", 是不能注册为商标, 或作为商标保护的。例如, 通用名为"苯磺酸氨氯地平片"的药品, 不同厂家生产, 可命名为"络活喜""兰迪""安内真"等不同的商品名。

🎧 **Task 4　Listen and complete. In pairs, listen to a dialogue between a nurse and a doctor, then fill the blanks in the prescription.**

听力 2.2

Juan Dela Cruz, M. D. 15th Street and Jones Ave. Holly, GA 22334 Phone# – 002 – 299 – 4598	
Patient Name (1) ＿＿＿＿＿	Date (2) ＿＿＿＿＿
Address (3) ＿＿＿＿＿	Age (4) ＿＿＿＿＿
R_X　Mefenamic Acid (5) ＿＿＿＿＿	mg #12
Sig: Take 1 (6) ＿＿＿＿＿ q4h for (7) ＿＿＿＿＿	days as needed for pain
J. D. Cruz M. D	Refill: (8) ＿＿＿＿＿
DEA#05368	

✎ Notes

1. "Mefenamic Acid" 是指药物"甲芬那酸", 具有解热、镇痛和消炎的作用, 可治疗发热、疼痛和炎症。

2. There is a prescription for her which is not completed. I wanted to check with you first.

护理人员在进行任何给药相关操作前, 都需要核实医嘱的信息, 如果发现医嘱信息不全, 需要和医生核对清楚后才可以执行。

3. Ms. Lucas is in good hands, isn't it? 卢卡斯女士得到了很好的照料, 不是吗?

句中的 "in good hands" 是指"受到很好的照料", 或在可靠（或内行）的人手里。

e. g. He had a minor heart attack. But he is in good hands.

他有点轻微心脏病发作, 不过医务人员会照顾好他的。

Task 5   Work in groups, use the following prescriptions and explain them to your partners. Swap roles and practice again.

Pt：Susan Diovan 40mg（pills） ii potid Dispense #60 Refill：1 time	Pt：Debby Glucophage 500mg（tabs） i po bid（pc） Dispense #60 Refill：3 times	Pt：Sally Zocor 5mg（capsules） i po qd（hs） Dispense #90 Refill：none

Communication Tips：

Communication in nursing is a central element of the healthcare system. When done right, everybody wins. Here are some strategies for effective communication within a multidisciplinary team.

1. Represent the nursing or midwifery perspective.

2. Consider the common goal – person – centered therapeutic care.

3. Remember you may not know everything about someone else's discipline – ask questions and be curious.

4. Show respect for each other's discipline.

5. Understand your colleague's role and scope of practice.

Listening and Speaking

Activity 2   Doing a Medication Check

Task 1   In pairs, match the 'five rights' (1 ~ 5) to their meanings (a ~ e).

1. the right patient	a. Check whether you are giving the medication by the correct route against Prescription Chart
2. the right drug	b. Check the patient's full name by checking the hospital label on the Prescription Chart and by checking the patient's ID band; check the patient's date of birth if necessary
3. the right dose	c. Check the frequency of medication is given and at what time
4. the right route	d. Check the medication you are giving against Prescription Chart is the one that was actually ordered
5. the right time	e. Check that the order is appropriate for the patient. Too much or too little of an adequately ordered medication can still cause issues for the patient

Notes

在西方国家，通常使用"五个准确"的药物核对制度，分别为"准确的病人；准确的药物；准确的给药途径；准确的给药时间；准确的剂量"，其所包含的具体信息和我国"三查七对"的信息是一致的。

Task 2　Listen to the conversation and complete the following extracts.

听力 2.3

Susan，a ward nurse，is looking for a nurse to help her with drug checks.

Lucy，（1）＿＿＿＿＿？I just need someone to help with drug check.

I am just（2）＿＿＿＿＿ and I can't leave it.

It is Ok. I'll see if Deon is（3）＿＿＿＿＿. Hi，Deon，（4）＿＿＿＿＿? Would you mind checking this insulin with me?

Susan. I'd love to help，but（5）＿＿＿＿＿ in work.

Hi，Joan，（6）＿＿＿＿＿? Can you do a drug check with me?

Thanks. I'll wait for you in the（7）＿＿＿＿＿.

Notes

1. I am just occupied with something. 我在忙着一些事情。

注意 "occupy" 的意思是 "keep busy with"，忙于做某事。

2. I'm up to my eyeballs in work. 我快要忙死了。

"up to my eyeballs" 表示 "工作太多，都堆积到视平线了"，意指太忙了，工作太繁重了。常见 "繁忙的" 的口语表达有 "snow under"，"flat out"，"run off one's feet" 等。

e. g. I'd love to help you，but I'm completely snowed under at the moment.

我很乐意帮助你，但我现在太忙了。

They're working flat out to finish on time. 他们正在加紧工作，想要准时完工。

He was run off his feet with jobs to do. 他忙得脚不沾地。

3. "Treating Room" 是指治疗室，一般护理人员会在治疗室进行药物的核对、检查和准备。

Task 3　Listen to the conversation and answer the following questions.

听力 2.4

Susan and Joan have gone to the treating room to get some medication for Mr. Yang.

1. What medication has the doctor prescribed for Mr. Yang?

＿＿＿＿＿＿＿＿＿＿

＿＿＿＿＿＿＿＿＿＿

2. Why does medicine need to be given 30 minutes before breakfast?

＿＿＿＿＿＿＿＿＿＿

＿＿＿＿＿＿＿＿＿＿

3. What information do the two nurses double check?

＿＿＿＿＿＿＿＿＿＿

＿＿＿＿＿＿＿＿＿＿

4. What do they have to do in the drug book?

＿＿＿＿＿＿＿＿＿＿

＿＿＿＿＿＿＿＿＿＿

5. How do Susan and Joan prevent medication administration errors?

＿＿＿＿＿＿＿＿＿＿

＿＿＿＿＿＿＿＿＿＿

✎ Notes

1. "MAR"是"medication administration record"的缩写，是指用药记录单。护理人员需要根据用药记录单的信息来核对药物和患者。

2. "Humulin N insulin"商品名为优泌林胰岛素，药品名为常规人胰岛素，主要适用于治疗需要采用胰岛素来维持正常血糖水平的糖尿病患者的治疗，属于高风险药物，所以该药物采用了双人核对的模式。

🎧 **Task 4** **Listen again. Match the strategies for the correct administration of medication to the rationales.**

听力 2.3

Strategies	Rationales
1. Susan and Joan validate carefully that MAR is consistent with the physician's order.	a. This is a safety check to ensure the right medication is selected.
2. Susan unlocks the medication cart.	b. It is to prove that the syringe contains the correct medication.
3. Susan and Joan retrieve medication to be given and compare the medication labels with MAR.	c. Errors in the transmission of intentions may occur between physician, pharmacy, and client's MAR.
4. Susan and Joan ensure the medication is indicated for the ordered route of administration and inspect the label for expiration date.	d. Limit access to and use special safeguards with "high alert" drugs.
5. Susan withdraws the correct amount of insulin from the ampoule and has Joan double check the calculation.	e. Different preparations of the same medication are used for different routes of administration. Out – of – date drugs can be less effective and risky.
6. Both Susan and Joan sign on the drug book.	f. Correct documentation can increase medication administration safety.
7. Joan will accompany Susan to give the injection of insulin.	g. It proves the patient has received the correct medication with the correct route.

✎ Notes

1. Susan and Joan validate carefully that MAR is consistent with the physician's order. 苏珊和琼仔细验证了用药记录单是否符合医师的医嘱。

"be consistent with"的意思是"与…一致"

e. g. His symptoms are not consistent with what he says.

他的症状和他描述的不一致。

2. Susan withdraws the correct amount of insulin from the ampoule.

苏珊从安瓿中抽出了正确剂量的胰岛素。

"withdraw"的意思是"移开，拿走，取出"

e. g. Nursing staffs are under enormous pressure when they withdraw life – sustaining measures from adult patients.

当护理人员从成年患者撤下维持生命的装置时，他们承受着巨大的压力。

3. Limit access to and use special safeguards with "hig – alert" drugs.

对于高危药物，需要限制访问权并使用特殊的保障措施。

"high – alert" drugs 和 "high – risk" drugs 都是指高危药物，在美国、英国等西方国家，界定为高危的药物都需要保存在在带有锁的药柜中，只有授权的医护人员才可以打开使用。

Task 5　Use Task 3 as a guide. In pairs, practice assisting with an insulin check. Use the following prompts to help you.

Medication Check Steps
Asking for assistance with a drug check
Verify the orders and the MAR
Unlock the cart and select the medication
Compare the medication label to the MAR
Check the expiry date
Withdraw the medication from the vial
Sign the name on the drug book
Take all the supplies to the ward

📖 Communication Tips：

Teamwork and collaboration are incredibly essential to the care for patients in a healthcare environment with various of health workers. Nurses should use different tips for working as part of a team.

Tips	Examples
Ask for assistance politely	I wonder if you could help me to check this medication.
Distribute the workload	Would you mind caring for Mr. Rob, and I'll look after his family members?
Offer alternative proposals	– Mr. Mike is refusing to take medicine. I don't know what to do. – He told me he hated the taste. It may be a good idea to talk with the doctor and get another brand.
Appreciate the contribution of other staff	I value your help, Anna. It was much easier to do this together.
Play an active part in creating a positive working environment	It is fantastic to be a part of the team. Does anyone need a hand since I've finished all my work?
Acknowledge when you're unable to offer a help	I'm up to my eyeballs in work. Can anyone else do it?

Listening and Speaking

Activity 3　Administering Medications

Task 1　Look at the pictures and explain the routes of drug administration.

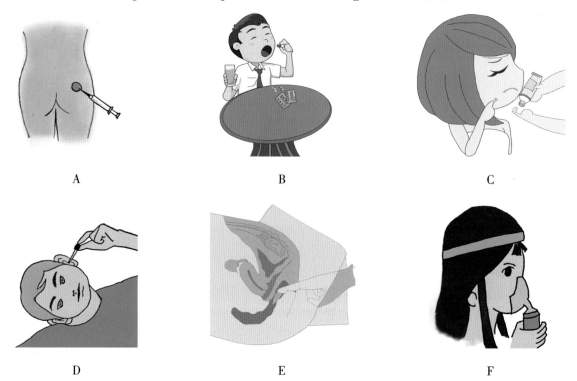

A　　　　　　　　　B　　　　　　　　　C

D　　　　　　　　　E　　　　　　　　　F

Notes

A route of drug administration is the path by which a drug is taken into the body. Routes of administration are generally classified by the location at which the drug is applied. Common examples include oral and intravenous administration. Routes can also be classified based on where the target of action is. Action maybe topical (local), enteral (system – wide effect, but delivered through the gastrointestinal tract), or parenteral (systemic action, but delivered by routes other than the GI tract).

给药途径是将药物吸收到体内的途径。给药途径通常根据药物的摄入的部位来分类。常见的途径有口服和静脉给药。给药途径也可以根据药物作用的目标部位来分类，作用可能是局部的，肠内的（全身作用，但通过胃肠道吸收）或肠胃外的（全身作用，但通过胃肠道以外的途径吸收）。

Task 2　Listen to the conversation and answer the following questions.

Susan and Joan have gone to the ward to administer a drug according to the order below.　　听力2.5

Patient：Xin Yang
Bed：4
DOB：10/05/1978
Rx：Humulin N insulin U – 500 Vial (500units/ml)
Sig：Administer 115units SC 30 minutes ac – breakfast – and 85units SC 30 minutes ac – lunch and evening meal.

1. What drug has the doctor prescribed for Mr. Yang?

_____

_____

2. What route do the nurses administer the drug? What's the time and the frequency of drug administration?

_____

_____

3. Do the nurses administer the medication safely? What strategies do they take to provide safe drug administration?

_____

_____

✎ Notes

1. The insulin helps to control your blood sugar and it's given via subcutaneous injection into the fatty tissue just below your skin.

胰岛素有助于控制您的血糖，给药方法通过皮下注射将药物注射到皮肤下方的脂肪组织。

护理人员在给药时，需要给患者进行健康教育，解释用药的目的和方法，有助于患者对于给药措施的理解和配合。

2. ID band，也被称为 "ID bracelet"，都是指 "身份腕带"。患者住院期间护理人员会给他们带上腕带，包含一些基本信息，方便医护人员对患者进行各种治疗和管理。

3. PDA Scanners，全称为 "personal data assistant scanners"，是一种医用手持的快速的数据采集智能设备，医护人员可通过 PDA 手持终端扫描患者腕带条码，确认患者的身份，实现智能化工作与管理。

4. Hypoglycemia may occur and is the most common side effect of insulin treatment. 胰岛素治疗最常见的副反应就是低血糖。

"Hypoglycemia" 是合成词指低血糖，由前缀 "hypo –" 表示 "below"，和词根 "glycemia" 表示 "sugar" 构成。

Task 3   Put the following stages of Susan and Joan's medication administration in the correct order. Listen again and check your answers.

听力 2.5

☐ Check the allergic history.
☐ Check the patient's ID number with the MAR and scan his ID band.
☐ Check the patient's name and DOB.
☐ Reassure the patient.
☐ Check the medication label with the MAR.
☐ Crosscheck the drug, the route, the dosage, and the time.
☐ Explain the purpose of medication administration.
☐ Countersign Medication Chart.

Notes

1. "allergic history" 是指 "过敏史"。胰岛素是一种生物制剂，绝大多数糖尿病患者注射后无不良反应，但是也有极少数出现过敏反应。所以注射胰岛素前护理人员必须要询问患者过敏史。

2. "reassure the patient" 是指 "安抚患者"。

If you reassure someone, you say or do things to make them stop worrying about something. 如果你安抚某人，你可以说或做一些事情让他们停止对某事的担忧。

e. g. **Patient**: I am worried that I'll be in a lot of pain after the operation.

Nurse: You'll have a PCA machine to use for any discomfort after the operation. Now, I will show you how to use it. And there are a variety of methods that can reduce pain after the procedure.

病人：我很担心手术后我会有很多的疼痛。

护士：在手术后，你可以使用止痛泵来减轻术后的任何不适。现在，我来教你如何使用它。而且还有很多方法可以减轻手术后的疼痛。

Task 4   **Listen to a conversation between a nurse Helen and Sum, a patient, and complete 1 ~ 9 in Sum's medication record.**

听力 2.6

Personal medication record			Patient：Sum		
Medication	**Reason for use**	**Form**	**Route**	**Dosage**	**Frequency**
Ciloxan	（1）_____	（2）_____	ophthalmic	（3）_____	Four times a day
（4）_____	Diabetes	capsule	（5）_____	One capsule a time	（6）_____
Benadryl	（7）_____	（8）_____	Oral	Two tablets a time	（9）_____

Notes

1. "general practitioner" 是指全科医生/家庭医生。在一些西方国家如英国，全科医生是最基层的医生，也是病人最先接触的医生，对病人的健康理念的干预效果最明显。患者生病，除了急症需要去急诊，通常会首先选择家庭医生而不是去专科门诊。

2. "affected eyes" 是指患眼。"affected" 意为 "患病的"。患侧可以表达为 "affected part"，患肢可以表达为 "affected limb"。

3. "over – the – counter medication" 是指非处方药物，简称为 "OTC" 药物。指消费者可自行在药店选用，以缓解轻度的短期症状及治疗轻微疾病的药品。

Task 5   **Use Task 4 as a guide, practice communicating with a patient when giving instructions to the patient about medication administration.**

Personal medication record Patient：＊＊					
Medication	**Reason for use**	**Form**	**Route**	**Dosage**	**Frequency**
Flonase	Rhinitis	Liquid	Nasal	Two sprays	Twice a day
Plendil	Hypertension	Pill	Oral	One pill a time on an empty stomach	Once a day
Dextromethorphan	Cough	Liquid	Oral	10 ~ 20mg one time	Every four hours

Communication Tips：

When you instruct a patient，you'd better use imperatives – take，don't take，you need to，etc. and simply explain the information.

e. g.

1. You need to take two capsules three times a day at bedtime.

2. Don't take more than two every six hours，and not more than eight tablets a time.

3. Only take this medicine by mouth.

Writing

If you are Nurse Susan in Activity 2 Task 4，please write the medication administration record after administering insulin to Mr. Yang. It should include patient's information，drug information，patient's reaction and some nursing considerations.

Proverbs and Sayings

◇ Save one life, you're a hero. Save 100 lives, you're a nurse.

救一个人，你是一个英雄；救一百个人，你是一位护士。

◇ Constant attention by a good nurse may be just as important as a major operation by a surgeon.

好护士的持续关注可和一个外科医生在大手术中的重要性一样。

◇ Do small things with great love.

用伟大的爱去做一些小事情。

书网融合……

听力材料 2.1　　　听力材料 2.2　　　听力材料 2.3

听力材料 2.4　　　听力材料 2.5　　　听力材料 2.6

Unit 3 Preventing Cross Infection

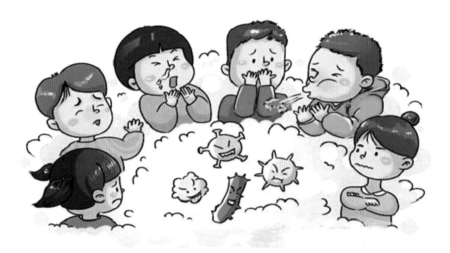

Learning Objectives

Reading part:

Be able to identify the details of infection control.

Listening and Speaking part:

1. Be able to identify and recognize personal preventive equipment.

2. Be able to correctly explain infection control to other healthcare providers, using effective communication strategies within a multidisciplinary team.

3. Be able to tell the process of using some personal preventive equipment.

4. Be able to identify and recognize specific information about preventing cross infections.

5. Be able to correctly introduce some information about doing a nucleic acid test, using effective communication strategies, and building a therapeutic relationship.

Writing part:

Be able to write a composition about the measures that are being taken to control COVID – 19 in China, using appropriate medical terminology, accurate grammar and punctuation.

Warm – up Exercises

China on May 13, 2021 inaugurated a new national administration of disease prevention and control, with its five major functions including formulating policies for the prevention and control of infectious diseases. The establishment of the administration signals the expansion of the roles of disease prevention and control agencies from preventing and containing diseases to comprehensively safeguarding and promoting the health of the entire population.

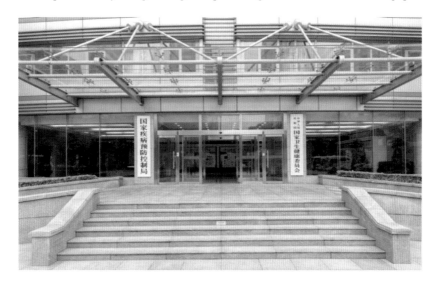

Work in pairs and discuss the following questions.

1. What are the risk factors for infection?

_____

_____

2. What are the effective ways to prevent infection?

_____

_____

3. Can you list the steps of washing hands?

_____

_____

Reading

阅读译文

Introduction to the Infection Control

Good health depends on good surroundings and the sense and practices of self – protection of the population. Techniques and practices that control or prevent the transmission of infection help to protect clients and healthcare workers from disease. Therefore, it is of great significance for the healthcare workers to take necessary measures to control and prevent infections and to sustain the safety of the environment and the health of clients and healthcare givers. The basic knowledge and aseptic techniques in preventing the spread of the infections such as cleaning, disinfection are the fundamental skills that the medical staff should acquire.

As we all know, germs are a part of everyday life and are found in our air, soil, water, and in and on our bodies. Some germs are helpful, others are harmful. Many germs live in and on our bodies without causing harm and some even help us to stay healthy. Only a small portion of germs are known to cause infection.

An infection occurs when germs enter the body, increase in number, resulting in the relevant diseases and the continuous spread of microorganisms outside.

The presence of infection depends on the following three elements:

Source of infecting microorganism: places where infectious agents (germs) live (e. g. sinks, surfaces, human skin)

Susceptible persons: a way for germs to enter the body

Means of transmission: a way germs are moved to the susceptible person

When the three elements exist simultaneously and there are chances for them to be related with each other, an infection occurs. Therefore, the healthcare workers can prevent the infection by taking infection prevention measures to break the chain of infection. We can isolate the source of infection, cut off the route of transmission, protect the susceptible persons to control the spread of infectious diseases.

After contacting with infection sources or before caring for the clients, the nurses should wash or disinfect hands to remove the dirt and adhered pathogens to avoid or reduce infection and cross infection. The healthcare workers use masks, gloves, shoe covers, isolation gowns, goggles, protective clothing, protective masks and other protective equipment at work. Among them, good hand hygiene is the most simple, efficient and cost - effective way to cut off the route of transmission of diseases transmitted by contact.

(372 words)

✎ Notes

1. The basic knowledge and aseptic techniques in preventing the spread of the infections such as cleaning, disinfection are the fundamental skills that the medical staff should acquire. 预防感染的基本知识和无菌技术如清洁和消毒是医务人员必须掌握的基本技能。

本句中 "disinfection" 应翻译为 "消毒"。前缀：dis - 在医学术语中是 "分离" 的意思，如 "dissection" 表示 "解剖，切开"。

e. g. In all cases, disinfection should be preceded by thorough cleaning. 在各种情况下，都应该通过彻底清洁进行消毒。

2. An infection occurs when germs enter the body, increase in number, resulting in the relevant diseases and the continuous spread of microorganisms outside. 所谓感染是病原体经过一定途径进入人体并不断繁殖，引起相应的病变并不断向外播散的过程。

本句中 "result in" 应翻译为 "导致，结果是"。

e. g. Fatigue and stress quickly result in a dull complexion. 疲劳和压力会很快导致肤色黯淡无光。

result in = lead to "导致，引起"，主语是原因，宾语是结果。

result from = because of "因 ... 而导致 ...", 宾语是原因，主语是结果。

e. g. The bad weather result in traffic jam. 坏天气导致了交通阻塞。

The traffic jam result from bad weather. 交通阻塞是由于坏天气。

3. Means of transmission: a way germs are moved to the susceptible person. 传播途径：细菌转移到易感人群的一种途径

本句中 "susceptible" 应翻译为 "易受外界影响的；易受感染的"。

e. g. Children are more susceptible than adults. 孩子比成人易受外界的影响。

4. After contacting with infection sources or before caring for the clients, the nurses should wash or disinfect hands to remove the dirt and adhered pathogens to avoid or reduce infection and cross – infection. 护理人员在接触感染源后或为患者进行护理操作前，均应洗手或消毒双手，以除去手上污垢及沾染的致病菌，避免或减少感染和交叉感染的发生率。

本句中"adhere"应翻译为"黏附"指用胶水、糨糊、黏结剂等粘贴，强调把某物紧紧地固定在另一物的表面上。

e. g. Abdominal tissues sometimes adhere after an operation. 手术之后腹部有时会出现粘连。

After – reading Exercises

Task 1   Match the words（1～10）with their proper meanings（a～j）.

1. Infection	a. 微生物
2. Transmission	b. 无菌的
3. Germ	c. 细菌
4. Microorganism	d. 易受感染地
5. Element	e. 口罩
6. Aseptic	f. 卫生
7. Susceptible	g. 传播
8. Mask	h. 感染
9. Goggles	i. 要素
10. Hygiene	j. 护目镜

Task 2   Complete the following sentences with a word or short phrase from the text.

1. Good health depends on good surroundings and the sense and practices of _____ of the population.

2. The basic knowledge and aseptic techniques in preventing the spread of the infections such as cleaning, _____ are the fundamental skills that the medical staff should acquire.

3. An _____ occurs when germs enter the body, increase in number, resulting in the relevant diseases and the continuous spread of microorganisms outside.

4. When the three elements exist _____ and there are chances for them to be related with each other, an infection occurs.

5. Among them, good hand _____ is the most simple, efficient and cost – effective way to cut off the route of transmission of diseases transmitted by contact.

Task 3   Work in pairs, discuss the following questions.

1. Do you think the infection control is important? Why?

_____

_____

_____

2. What are the three basic elements of infection?

____

____

____

Listening and Speaking

Activity 1　Preventing Cross Infection among Medical Staff

Task 1　The following equipment are commonly used on personal prevention. Work in pairs, match the terms (1 ~ 10) with English expressions (a ~ j).

1. 医用外科口罩	a. isolation gown
2. 护目镜	b. disinfectant
3. 隔离衣	c. surgical mask
4. 消毒剂	d. disposable medical gloves
5. 一次性医用手套	e. goggles
6. 蚊帐	f. ultraviolet lamp
7. 单间病室	g. single room
8. 无菌持物钳	h. sterile rubber gloves
9. 无菌乳胶手套	i. sterile transfer forceps
10. 紫外线灯	j. mosquito net

Notes

Personal protective equipment refers to the personal protective equipment provided in the process of labor production to protect workers from or reduce the injury of accidents and occupational hazards, which plays a direct role in protecting human body.

个人防护用品是指在劳动生产过程中使劳动者免遭或减轻事故伤害和职业危害因素的伤害而提供的个人保护装备，直接对人体起到保护作用。

听力 3.1

Task 2　Listen to the conversation and complete the following extracts.

Susan, a nurse, is explaining to John, a new nurse, how to prevent cross infection.

John: Good morning, Susan. Since I am a freshman and work in the department of (1) ____________, I am worried about to get infected someday.

Susan: All right. You should not have excessive anxiety. Just do proper (2) ________________ to avoid or reduce infection and cross infection.

John: What do you mean by cross infection?

Susan: Cross infection generally refers to the mutual infection caused by various ways between patients or between patients and medical care in medical units.

John：Does this happen often?

Susan：That depends. The main causes of cross infection are related to the lack of protection awareness of medical staff, the disinfection and isolation management system of hospitals and wards, and the unreasonable layout of wards in hospitals.

John：We should pay more attention in daily life.

Susan：That's right. It's not too much to (3) _____ the importance of prevention.

John：What are the common ways of infection?

Susan：The main ways of cross infection in hospital are air, (4) _____, contact, injection, infusion and so on.

John：And anything else?

Susan：If the (5) _____ or the medical instruments are not strictly disinfected, cross – infection such as hepatitis B or C can be caused during injection, dental visits, or gastroscopy.

John：Oh, that's a very serious public health issue.

※ Notes

1. infectious disease 是"传染病"，英文解释是指"a disease transmitted only by a specific kind of contact，"即一种必须通过某一种特殊途径进行传播的疾病。

e. g. Sufferers from the infectious disease are isolated. 感染到这种传染病的人被隔离起来。

2. overemphasize 是"过分强调"，英文解释是"place special or excessive emphasis on."

e. g. Some students tend to overemphasize the influence of objective forces when they fail some subjects. 有些学生过分强调考试不及格的客观原因。

Task 3　Put the following stages of washing hands in the correct order. Work in pairs and check your answers.

(　) a. Rub right thumb in the fisted left palm. Then exchange the position of hands.

(　) b. Rub the fingertips in left palm. Exchange the position of hands.

(　) c. Scrub soap on palms with a circular motion and rub the hands to make foam.

(　) d. Turn on water using elbow or foot controls. Rinse hands thoroughly under running water from fingertips to elbows and then dry them.

(　) e. Rub palmar side of the fingers with the palm of another hand.

(　) f. Flex fingers of left hand in right palm, and rub with right palm. Then exchange the position of hands.

(　) g. Interlace fingers to friction. Cover and rub the back of left hand with right palm. Exchange the position of hands.

※ Notes

1. Rub the fingertips in left palm. 右手指尖在左掌心揉搓。

"rub"在这里的意思是"揉搓"。

e. g. He rubbed his arms and stiff legs. 他揉了揉自己的胳膊和僵硬的双腿。

Rub the cream in with a circular motion. 转着圈将乳霜揉进去。

2. Scrub soap on palms with a circular motion and rub the hands to make foam. 在手掌上转圈擦洗肥皂，用手揉成泡沫。

"scrub" 是指"擦洗，刷洗"。

e. g. Surgeons began to scrub their hands and arms with soap and water before operating. 外科医生们在手术前开始用肥皂和水清洗他们的手和手臂。

3. Rinse hands thoroughly under running water from fingertips to elbows and then dry them. 在自来水下彻底冲洗双手，从指尖到肘部，然后干燥。

"rinse" 在这里的意思是"指用清水冲洗、清洗、冲掉皂液"。

e. g. Make sure you rinse all the soap out. 一定要把皂液冲洗干净。

"running water" 意思是"自来水；流水，活水"。

e. g. Rinse the vegetables under cold running water. 用凉的自来水清洗这些蔬菜。

听力 3.2

Task 4 Listen to the conversation and complete the following extracts.

Susan, a nurse, is explaining to John, a new nurse, how to wear an isolation gown.

Susan：John, Here you are. Put it on.

John：Oh, What's this?

Susan：To protect hospital personnel and avoid cross infection, we need to wear (1) _____ when caring for isolated clients.

John：Could you tell me the procedures?

Susan：First, you take out an isolation gown. The (2) _____ side should toward you. Insert the hand into one sleeve, then (3) _____ another hand into another sleeve. Button up the neckline button and the sleeve buttons. Hold one side of the gown to the front. Hold another side of the gown the same way. Make (4) _____ of the two edge of the gown. Overlap the gown on the back. (5) _____ the girdle.

John：Thank you.

Notes

1. We need to wear isolation gown when caring for isolated clients. 在护理隔离患者时，我们需要穿隔离衣。

"isolate" 意思是"（使）隔离，孤立"；"isolation" 意思是"隔离，隔离状态"。

e. g. Patients will be isolated from other people for between three days and one month after treatment. 治疗结束后，病人将与其他人隔离 3 天到 1 个月的时间。

They live in an isolated area and have no neighbors. 他们住在一个隔离区，没有邻居。

2. Overlap the gown on the back. 在后背，将隔离衣重叠交叉对齐。

"overlap" 意思是"重叠，交叠"。

e. g. The needs of patients invariably overlap. 病人的需求总有一些是一致的。

Task 5 Put the following stages of removing isolation gown in the correct order. Work in pairs and check your answers.

(　) a. Pull up the sleeves and tuck them under the sleeves of arms.

(　) b. Pull the other contaminated sleeve with the sleeve‐covered hand.

(　) c. Pull down the clean inside of the gown with the clean hand.

(　) d. Untie the girdle and make a loose knot in the front part of gown.

(　) e. Lift the sleeves, make parallel of the edges of the gown and hang the gown on the hoop.

🛠 Notes

"contaminate" 意思是 "污染，弄脏"。

e. g. contaminated blood/food/soil 受到污染的血液 / 食物 / 土壤

Her infection was traced to contaminated food. 她的感染被查出是由受到污染的食物所致。

👥 Communication Tips：

Since most patients are outsiders in medicine, unclear, incorrect and infeasible ideas are common and understandable. Nurses should patiently explain to patients with experience and data. It is better to speak in plain language and clear and vivid facts. So, it is necessary to clarify some inaccurate, infeasible, even biased and wrong ideas.

Patient：Nurse, since the COVID - 19 has subsided in China and the vaccination is of little significance. I don't want to get vaccinated.

Nurse：It is very important to get vaccinated. Under the background that the global COVID - 19 is still epidemic, our country's COVID - 19 prevention and control measures are effective and the domestic risk of infection is relatively low, but the risk of imported and transmitted infections still exists. So, vaccination is everyone's responsibility.

Listening and Speaking

Activity 2　Doing a Nucleic Acid Test

Task 1　The following terms are related to 2019 - nCoV. Work in pairs, match the terms（1 ~ 10）with English expressions（a ~ j）.

1. 冠状病毒	a. pneumonia
2. 肺炎	b. vaccine
3. 疫苗	c. incubation period
4. 潜伏期	d. virus carrier
5. 病毒携带者	e. coronavirus
6. 咽拭子	f. confirmed case
7. 抗体	g. mobile cabin hospital
8. 确诊病例	h. throat swab
9. 疑似病例	i. suspected case
10. 方舱医院	j. antibody

🛠 Notes

2019 novel Coronavirus（2019 - nCoV）was named by WHO in January 2020. The common signs of coronavirus infection include respiratory symptoms, fever, cough, shortness of breath and dyspnea. In more severe cases, infection can lead to pneumonia, severe acute respiratory syndrome, renal failure, and even death.

新型冠状病毒（2019 - nCoV），于 2020 年 1 月被世界卫生组织（WHO）命名。人感染了冠状病毒后常见体征有呼吸道症状、发热、咳嗽、气促和呼吸困难等。在较严重病例中，感染可导致肺炎、严重急性呼吸综合征、肾衰竭，甚至死亡。

🎧 **Task 2　Listen to the conversation and complete the following extracts.**

听力 3.3

Susan，a nurse，is doing a physical assessment and collecting data from a patient.

Susan：Good morning. What can I do for you?

Patient：Good morning, nurse. I have a terrible headache.

Susan：All right. Tell me how it got started?

Patient：I had a (1) _____ nose yesterday. And I have a (2) _____ throat now.

Susan：Don't worry. Let me give you an examination. Open your mouth and say "ah".

Patient：Ah...

Susan：Good. Now put your tongue out. Look, your throat is (3) _____. And I will take a temperature immediately.

Patient：Thanks.

Susan：Time is up. Please take out the (4) _____.

Patient：Here you are.

Susan：Oh, your temperature is 37.6℃. You've got a fever.

Patient：Oh, no. Does it mean I've got novel coronavirus pneumonia? What should I do next?

Susan：Don't worry. I will take you to the isolation room now. And you will do a (5) _____ test.

Patient：OK. I will follow your advice.

Nurse：The result will come out in six hours. During this time, you should wait in this isolation room and wear the mask all the time.

✂ **Notes**

1. Does it mean I've got novel coronavirus pneumonia? 这是不是意味着我得了新冠肺炎啊？

"pneumonia"和"pneumonitis"均指肺炎。严格讲，"Pneumonia is a type of pneumonitis because the infection cause inflammation"，即"pneumonia"指的是传染造成的肺炎。

2. In the early stage of the novel coronavirus infection, the main symptoms arelow-grade fever and general fatigue. Some patients will have mild cough symptoms.

新型冠状病毒感染的前期，最主要的症状是低热，全身乏力，有些病人会出现轻度咳嗽的症状。

发热的程度分为低热、中等热、高热和超高热，用英文分别表示为"mild/low-grade fever""moderate grade fever""high-grade fever"和"hyperpyrexia"。

🎧 **Task 3　Listen to the conversation and answer the following questions.**

听力 3.4

Nurse Linda is doing a nucleic acid test for a patient.

（1）What is a nucleic acid test?

_____

_____

（2）Why does the nurse require the patient to tilt the head back slightly?

_____

_____

（3）List the steps of doing a nucleic acid test.

_____

_____

✎ Notes

The substance of nucleic acid detection is the nucleic acid of virus. Nucleic acid detection is to find out whether there is foreign virus nucleic acid in respiratory tract samples, blood or feces of patients to determine whether they are infected by new coronavirus. Therefore, once the detection of nucleic acid "positive", it can prove that there is a virus in the patient's body.

核酸检测的物质是病毒的核酸。核酸检测是为了查明患者的呼吸道标本、血液或粪便中是否存在外来病毒的核酸，以确定他们是否感染了新冠状病毒。因此一旦检测为核酸"阳性"，即可证明患者体内有病毒存在。

Task4　Put the following stages of doing a nucleic acid test in the correct order. Work in pairs and check your answers.

（　）a. Sample submission for inspection.

（　）b. Collect secretions.

（　）c. Secretion retention.

（　）d. Fluorescence PCR nucleic acid detection.

（　）e. Nucleic acid extraction.

（　）f. Issue a nucleic acid test report.

Task 5　Use Task 3 as a guide, practice communicating with a patient when doing nucleic acid testing.

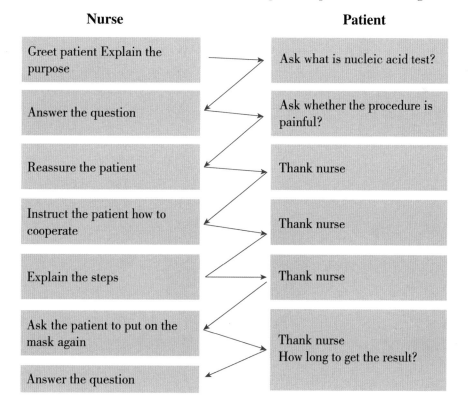

Communication Tips：

Timely rhetorical question

It is applicable to repeat and verify the patient's speech. This kind of method is used to verify the authenticity of the conversation with patients and ensure the accuracy of data collection.

Patient：Nurse, I want to take my blood pressure.

Nurse：All right. Please sit down to have a rest for a while. Please straighten the tested limb and slightly abduct the palm upward. Your blood pressure is normal, is there anything uncomfortable with you?

Patient：Oh, Great! I feel much better than before.

Nurse：You just said you feel much better than before, don't you?

Listening and Speaking

Activity 3   Informing the Interventions about Preventing Cross Infections

Task 1   Look at the pictures and name them.

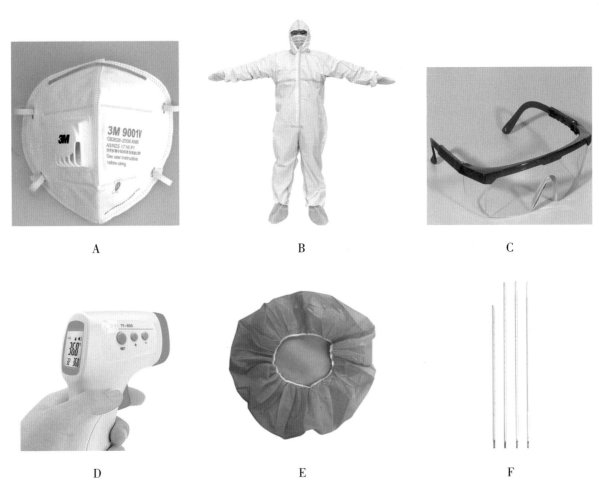

A   B   C

D   E   F

⚒ Notes

Cross infection is the phenomenon that pathogens from natural hosts infect or transmit to non – natural hosts. It refers to the local tissue and systemic inflammatory reaction caused by the invasion of bacteria, viruses, fungi, parasites and other pathogens into the human body.

交叉感染是天然宿主的病原体感染或传递给非天然宿主的现象，是指细菌、病毒、真菌、寄生虫等病原体侵入人体所引起的局部组织和全身性炎症反应。

Task 2　Listen to the conversation and answer the following questions.

听力3.5

Danny, a family member of the patient, is talking with Susan, a nurse.

Susan：Good morning, Danny. Are you the husband of Julie who is in bed 15?

Danny：Good morning, Susan. Yes, I am her husband.

Susan：Since Julie is admitted to the department of (1) _____ disease, I need to explain some rules you should follow.

Danny：OK.

Susan：The hospital is a (2) _____ area where people gather. It needs the joint cooperation of medical staff, medical auxiliary staff and other personnel, like you, the caregivers.

Danny：I will work with you.

Susan：First of all, family members are not allowed to (3) _____ the patients when they stay in the department of infectious disease.

Danny：Can we visit her during the visiting hours?

Susan：Generally, it is not allowed to pay a visit to contagious patients. If it is necessary, the visitors should wear a (4) _____ isolation gown and isolation shoes, wear a (5) _____, and wash hands with sterile water after the visit.

Danny：It is ok. As far as she can make a full (6) _____, we would like do anything.

Susan：Wish your wife a speedy recovery.

⚒ Notes

1. "sterile" 无菌的，英文解释是 "free of or using methods to keep free of pathological microorganisms."

e. g. The doctor kept his instruments sterile. 这位医生的器具是消过毒的。

2. As far as she can make a full recovery, we would like do anything. 只要她能痊愈，我们愿意做任何事。

"recovery" 的意思是 "愈合"。当一个患者从疾病状态完全恢复到健康时，我们就说这个患者痊愈了，可以用 "The patient makes a good/full/complete recovery" 来表达。

Task 3　Listen again and answer the following questions.

听力3.5

1. Is the hospital a safe place where people gather?

_____

_____

2. Is it allowed for the family members to pay a visit for the patients in the department of infectious disease?

_____

_____

3. What procedure should visitors take if they pay a visit to contagious patients?

_____

_____

Notes

Chances of contamination are higher if people do not wash their hands after touching objects, as it's possible they could be infected by rubbing their eyes or scratching their nose and mouth. Children, the elderly and other people whose immunity is relatively weak can easily get infected in this way.

如果人们在接触物体后不洗手，感染的机会就会增高，因为他们可能会通过揉眼睛或抓鼻子和嘴巴而被感染。儿童、老人等免疫力较弱的人，更容易通过接触被污染的物品而感染。

听力 3.6

Task 4   Listen to a nurse making a health education about preventing COVID – 19 in the community and fill the blanks.

Hi, everyone. I am a (1) _____ nurse, Deon. I'd like to make a short speech about how to prevent COVID – 19 in the community. Thanks for your attention in advance. In case of preventing COVID – 19 spread in your community, please follow the instructions. Wash your hands well and often. Use hand (2) _____ when you're not near soap and water. Try not to (3) _____ your face. Wear a face mask when you go out. Follow your community guidelines for staying home. When you do go out in public, leave at least 6 (4) _____ of space between you and others. Don't worry if you cannot remember all the (5) _____. Here are some brochures with WHO's recommendations on for preventing (6) _____. Feel free to take them home.

Notes

Use hand sanitizer when you're not near soap and water. 当附近没有肥皂和水源时，使用手消毒液。

"sanitizer" 是指 "消毒剂"。It is a substance or product that is used to reduce or eliminate pathogenic agents on surfaces. 它是指减少或清除物品表面的病原微生物的物品。"disinfectant" 也可翻译为 "消毒剂"。It is a chemical substance or compound used to inactivate or destroy microorganisms on surfaces. 它是一种化学物质或化合物，用于灭活或破坏物体表面上的微生物。他们的区别是 "disinfectant" 可杀灭全部或绝大多数微生物，而 "sanitizer" 不能杀灭全部微生物。

Task 5   Work in groups, use the following sentences to make a health education about preventing COVID – 19. Swap roles and practice again.

> Wash your hands well and often.
>
> Use hand sanitizer when you're not near soap and water.
>
> Try not to touch your face.
>
> Wear a face mask when you go out.
>
> Follow your community guidelines for staying home.
>
> When you do go out in public, leave at least 6 feet of space between you and others.

Communication Tips：

Clarification

In the later stage of explanation, a very important skill of intention is to verify and clarify the patient's understanding, avoid ineffective communication, and even lead to misunderstanding or disputes. Let the patient speak out the information they understand and see if they really understand it clearly.

Nurse: Good afternoon, Mr. Li. How are you feeling now? Do you still have pain in your chest?

Patient: No, there is no more pain, but I feel a little tight in my chest. I also feel dizzy when I stand up.

Nurse: Your EEG shows that you have coronary heart disease. Your attack was brought on by an insufficient blood supply to the heart.

Patient: Will it happen again?

Nurse: If you follow the doctor's instructions, perhaps it will not happen.

Patient: That's fine. Thank you. By the way, could you tell me something special I should do in my daily life?

Nurse: Yes. Pay attention to your diet. Your meals should be frequent but small in quantity. However, you must not forget that you should take plenty of vegetables and fruits.

Patient: I know.

Nurse: In order to make sure that I have explained it clearly, please tell me what we talked about in your own words?

Writing

In recent years, everywhere around the globe is buzzing with talk on how to control the rapid spread of the coronavirus. China's COVID – 19 has been effectively controlled and achieved a stage victory. Please describe the measures that are being taken to control Coronavirus in China.

Proverbs and Sayings

✧ Treatment is more about restoring the peace of mind than about producing a cure.
医学治疗的宗旨不只是要治疗疾病，更要助人心安。

✧ A good healthy body is worth more a crown in gold.
健康的身体贵于黄金铸成的皇冠。

✧ Prevention comes before treatment.
预防胜于治疗。

书网融合……

听力材料3.1　　听力材料3.2　　听力材料3.3　　听力材料3.4　　听力材料3.5　　听力材料3.6

Unit 4　Preparing Patients for Radiology

PPT

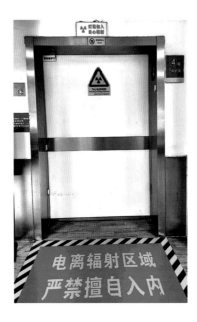

Learning Objectives

Reading part：

Be able to identify the details of the imaging tests in hospital.

Listening and Speaking part：

1. Be able to identify and recognize specific information on imaging tests in hospital.

2. Be able to correctly explain the method and importance of imaging examination in hospital to other healthcare providers, using effective communication strategies within a multidisciplinary team.

3. Be able to check the consistency of patient information and doctor's order, when patients need imaging examination.

4. Be able to communicate with other nurses in the process of patient information checking and doctor's order checking, and use communication skills as part of the team.

5. Be able to explain the cause and precautions of imaging examination correctly according to the doctor's order and the patient's condition, and establish the treatment relationship by using effective communication strategies.

Writing part：

Be able to write imaging examination records with appropriate medical terms, accurate grammar and punctuation symbols.

Warm – up Exercises

Lucy is a nurse. One of her tasks is to explain the purpose, methods and differences of various imaging examinations to patients. Can you help her label different types of imaging tests and describe their main functions?

Angiogram	CT – scan	Mammogram	MRI	Ultrasound	X – ray

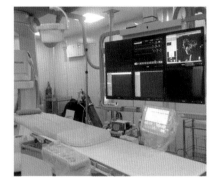

A _____

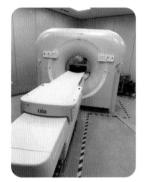

B _____

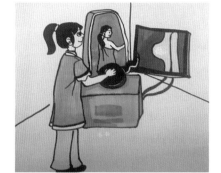

C _____

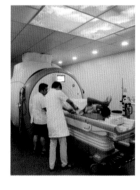

D _____

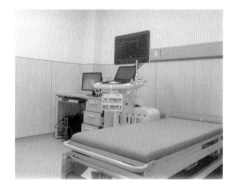

E _____

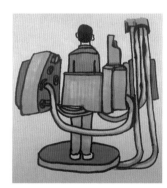

F _____

Reading

阅读译文

Introduction to the Imaging Tests in Hospital

Imaging tests provide pictures of the body's interior—of the whole body or part of it. Imaging helps doctors diagnose a disorder, determine how severe the disorder is, and monitor people after the disorder is diagnosed.

Imaging tests may use the following:

✦ Radiation, as in X – rays, angiography, computed tomography (CT), and radionuclide scanning, including positron emission tomography (PET)

✦ Sound waves, as in ultrasonography

✦ Magnetic fields, as in magnetic resonance imaging (MRI)

✦ Substances that are swallowed, injected, or inserted to highlight or outline the tissue or organ to be examined (called contrast agents)

X – rays

X – rays are high – energy radiation waves that can penetrate most substances (to varying degrees). For conventional X – ray imaging, a person is positioned so that the body part to be evaluated is between the X – ray source and a device that records the image. An X – ray beam is aimed at the body part to be evaluated. Different tissues block different amounts of the X – rays, depending on the tissue's density. The denser the tissue, the more X – rays it blocks and the whiter the image.

CT

In computed tomography (CT), which used to be called computed axial tomography (CAT), an X – ray source and X – ray detector rotate around a person. People should wear clothing that has no metallic buttons, snaps, zippers, or other metal in it over the area to be scanned and should remove any jewelry. Such items are not dangerous but may block X – rays and distort the image. For CT, people may be given a radiopaque contrast agent . Contrast agents are substances that can be seen on X – rays and help distinguish one tissue from another. The contrast agents may be injected into a vein, taken by mouth, or inserted through the anus. The contrast agents used depends on what type of test is done and which body part is being evaluated.

Ultrasonography

Ultrasonography uses high – frequency sound (ultrasound) waves to produce images of internal organs and other tissues. No X – rays are used, so there is no radiation exposure during an ultrasonography. Ultrasonography is painless, relatively inexpensive, and considered very safe, even during pregnancy. Usually, the examiner places thick gel on the skin over the area to be examined to ensure good sound transmission. A handheld transducer is placed on the skin and moved over the area to be evaluated. After the test, most people can resume their usual activities immediately.

MRI

In magnetic resonance imaging (MRI), a strong magnetic field and very high frequency radio waves are used to produce highly detailed images. For MRI, a person lies on a motorized table that is moved into the narrow interior of a large tubular scanner, which produces a strong magnetic field. Examiners can change how various tissues appear on a scan by varying the radio wave pulses, the strength and direction of the magnetic field, and other factors.

(476 words)

✕ Notes

1. Imaging tests provide pictures of the body's interior—of the whole body or part of it. 影像学检查提供全身或部分身体内部的图像。

interior 翻译为 "内部，里面"。英文解释为 "the internal or inner part of a thing"，即物体的内部或里面。

e. g. The endocardium is the thin membrane that lines the interior of the heart. 心内膜是排列在心脏内部的薄膜。

2. Imaging helps doctors diagnose a disorder, determine how severe the disorder is, and monitor people after the disorder is diagnosed.

影像学检查可以帮助医生诊断疾病，确定疾病的严重程度，并在疾病诊断后监测患者。

monitor 翻译为 "监测"，也可译为 "监护仪"。

e. g. The heart monitor shows low levels of consciousness.

心脏监控器显示患者处于低意识水平。

3. contrast agent 指造影剂，是为增强影像观察效果而注入（或服用）到人体组织或器官的化学制品。这些制品的密度高于或低于周围组织，形成的对比用某些器械显示图像。如 X 线观察常用的碘制剂、硫酸钡等。

After – reading Exercises

Task 1   Match the medical imaging tests （1 ~ 6） to the usages （a ~ f）.

1. Angiogram	a. Take a picture of the breast.
2. CT scan	b. A way of ultrasonic examination gives a 3 – D image of the body.
3. Mammogram	c. A high – energy radiation wave that can penetrate most substances.
4. MRI	d. Use a magnetic field to take pictures of the body.
5. B – ultrasound examination	e. Take an image of the blood vessels.
6. X – ray	f. Use X – rays and computers to produce images of a cross – section of your body.

Task 2   Complete the following sentences with a word or short phrase from the text.

1. Imaging tests may use the following： _____ , _____ , MRI, B – ultrasound, angiogram, mammogram, ultrasound, etc.

2. Different tissues block different amounts of the X – rays, depending on the tissue's _____ . The denser the tissue, the more X – rays it blocks and the _____ the image.

3. _____ are substances that can be seen on X – rays and help distinguish one tissue from another.

4. No X – rays are used, so there is no radiation exposure during an _____ .

5. For _____ , a person lies on a motorized table that is moved into the narrow interior of a large tubular scanner, which produces a strong magnetic field.

Task 3   In pairs, discuss the following questions.

1. Do you think imaging tests in hospitals are essential? Why?

_____

_____

2. Why is protection required during imaging examination?

_____

_____

_____

Listening and Speaking

Activity 1   Getting CT Scan Consent for IV Contrast Injection

Task 1   Match the terms (1 ~ 7) to their meanings (a ~ g).

1. Complications	a. hypersensitivity reaction to a particular allergen
2. Allergy	b. the act of watching sb./sth. carefully for a period of time, especially to learn sth.
3. Observation	c. Patients understand and approve their condition and the diagnosis and treatment plan made by doctors
4. Contrast agent	d. Chemicals injected (or taken) into human tissues or organs to enhance imaging observation
5. Diabetes mellitus	e. Metabolic diseases characterized by hyperglycemia
6. Informed consent	f. Also known as toxic diffuse goiter, it is an autoimmune disease with hypermetabolism and goiter
7. Hyperthyroidism	g. One disease causes another disease or symptom in the course of development. The latter is a complication of the former

Notes

A patient consent form is a document with important information about a medical procedure or treatment, a clinical trial, or genetic testing. It also includes information on possible risks and benefits. If a person chooses to participate in the treatment, procedure, trial, or testing, he or she signs the form to give official consent.

患者知情同意书是包含有关医疗程序或治疗、临床试验或基因检测的重要信息的文件。它还包括有关可能的风险和受益的信息。如果一个人选择参加治疗、程序、试验或测试，他要在表格上签名以表示正式同意。

Task 2   In pairs, read the following consent form and answer the questions.

Consent Form for Enhanced CT – scan		
The possible minor side effects and complications include but are not exclusive of flushing of the skin, nausea, etc. More severe side effects occur less often and involve lowering of the blood pressure, etc. Medications and personnel are here to treat any of these events.		
Please answer all of the following questions：	Yes	No
Do you have any history of allergy to iodine, foods, drugs, or medications? If yes, to what substances are you allergic? ＿＿＿＿＿＿		
Do you take Glucophage / Metformin? Check BUN and Creatinine to see if it has returned to baseline after the procedure. BUN ＿＿＿＿＿ Creatinine ＿＿＿＿＿ Date ＿＿＿＿＿		

续表

Do you have any historyof： Hypertension　Asthma　Diabetes　Seizures　Tumors　Myeloma Kidney Disease　Aneurysm　Heart Disease	
The examination has been explained to me including the benefits and alternative examinations. All questions have been answered to my satisfaction. I understand the above and consent to and agree with having this examination.	
Patient：	Family members（guardians）：
Doctor：	Date：

1. What examination will the patient have?

_____

_____

2. What kind of information will the nurse collect before an enhanced CT scan?

_____

_____

3. Why does a patient need to sign an informed consent form before an enhanced CT scan?

_____

_____

✖ Notes

1. Do you take Glucophage / Metformin?

你服用过格华止（抗糖尿病药）或二甲双胍吗？

A patient is to be off these medications for 48 hours after IV contrast administration.

患者需在静脉注射造影剂后 48 小时内停止服用这些药物。

2. Do you have any history of allergy to iodine, foods, drugs or medication?

是否有对碘、食物或药物的过敏史？

在进行增强 CT 检查前需询问过敏史，如食物过敏史、药物过敏史、是否对碘过敏等。

3. Do you have any history of kidney disease? 你以前得过肾脏方面的疾病吗？

由于碘对比剂主要经过肾脏排泄，若存在肾功能损害，影响造影剂的排出，可选择其他方法进行检查。

🎧 Task 3　Listen to the conversation and complete the following sentences.

1. There will be some discomfort and allergic reactions. For example, _____ , nausea, _____ , rash and so on.

2. Are you _____ to any food or drugs?

3. I have been _____ type 2 diabetes for many years.

听力 4.1

4. I'll _____ the radiologist knows before the enhanced CT – scan.

5. There are some _____ you need to take. Firstly, after the examination, sit for 30 minutes and _____ whether there is any discomfort. Secondly, after the examination, you need to drink more water.

Notes

1. nausea 恶心；vomiting 呕吐；

e. g. Minor toxicities of this drug include nausea and vomiting.

这种药的轻微毒性反应包括恶心和呕吐。

2. drink more water 译为 "多喝水"，可以帮助加速造影剂的排出。

3. make sure 译为 "确保，务必"

We make sure our clients get the best that money can buy.

我们确保客户买到最好的产品。

Task 4 Listen to the conversation again and answer the questions.

听力 4.1

1. What corresponding side effects does CT examination have?

_____

_____

2. What are the precautions for CT examination?

_____

_____

3. Does the patient have a history of hypertension, kidney disease and heart disease?

_____

_____

Notes

1. side effects 翻译为 " (药物的) 副作用；意外的连带后果"。

e. g. This drug is known to have adverse side effects.

众所周知，这种药具有不良副作用。

2. precautions 翻译为 "注意事项"。

此外，还可译为 "预防措施"。

e. g. You must take all reasonable precautions to protect yourself and your family.

你必须采取一切合理的预防措施，保护自己和家人。

Task 5 Use Task 2 and Task 3 as a guide. Make conversations in pairs. Student A, a nurse, ask questions to fill out the consent form. Student B, a patient, use patient 1 information to answer the nurse's questions. Exchange roles and practice again using patient 2 information.

THE EDWARD HOSPITAL
CT – SCAN CONSENT FOR IV CONTRAST INJECTION FORM

Patient 1　information
Name：Mr Michael Cole
Past Medical History：Heart disease（3 years）, Kidney disease
Allergies：Allergy to Eggs and animal hair
CT scan venography experience：No
Diabetes medications：Metformin
Pregnancy：N/A
Breastfeeding：N/A

Patient 2　information
Name：Ms Brianna
Past Medical History：Kidney disease（5 years）, diabetes, asthma（3 years）
Allergies：No
CT scan venography experience：Yes
Diabetes medications：Insulin
Pregnancy：No
Breastfeeding：No

Notes

N/A 是 Not Applicable 的缩写，意思为"不适用，不可用"。

在 Patient 1 的信息中，因该患者为男性，所以怀孕、母乳喂养不适用于该患者。而 Patient 2 的信息中，该患者是女性，用的是 No，说明该患者目前没有怀孕、母乳喂养的状况。

Communication Tips：

Nurses must always ask patients for their consent and permission before a procedure. Consent is a crucial component of establishing a respectful and trusting relationship with your patient—one that improves satisfaction, adherence, and ultimately, outcomes. Here are some expressions the nurses can use to obtain consent.

e. g. Would you mind…?

Could I possibly …?

Is it all right if you …?

Do you think you could…?

Is that ok…?

Listening and Speaking

Activity 2　Preparing a Patient for CT Scan

Task 1　Discuss three types of CT scan in pairs, and match（A ~ C）with（1 ~ 3）.

A——Plain CT

B——Enhanced CT

C——Image result for Cisternography CT

CT diagnostic classification	
1	It is X – ray computed tomography（CT）using radiocontrast. Radiocontrasts for X – ray CT are, in general, iodine – based types. This is useful to highlight structures such as blood vessels that otherwise would be difficult to delineate from their surroundings.

续表

2	A computerized tomography (CT) scan combines a series of X – ray images taken from different angles around your body and uses computer processing to create cross – sectional images (slices) of the bones, blood vessels and soft tissues inside your body. CT scan images provide more – detailed information than plain X – rays do.
3	Computed tomography (CT) cisternography is an imaging technique used to diagnose CSF rhinorrhea or CSF otorrhea (CSF leaks), as CT allows the assessment of the bones of the base of the skull.

✎ Notes

1. CT 检查一般包括平扫 CT (Plain CT)、增强 CT (Enhanced CT) 和脑池造影 CT (Image result for Cisternography CT)。

2. 平扫 CT (Plain CT) 和增强 CT (Enhanced CT) 区别：

(1) 平扫 CT 不需注射对比剂，增强 CT 扫描需手臂静脉注射对比剂后进行 CT 成像，可提高病灶检出率；

(2) 病灶性质不同强化模式也不同，增强 CT 对病灶的定性有所提高，一般疾病可根据增强 CT 表现做出准确诊断；

(3) 增强 CT 可较好了解恶性肿瘤患者分期、浸润程度、有无淋巴转移、脏器转移等；

(4) 增强 CT 可显示血管病变，血管堵塞情况，更好指导临床治疗。

🎧 **Task 2　Listen to the conversation and complete the following extracts.**

听力 4.2

At 9 o'clock tomorrow morning, Mr. Bob needs to have (1) ＿＿＿＿＿＿. Before the CT scan, Mr. Bob need to take off the (2) ＿＿＿＿＿＿, including jewelry, eyeglasses, dentures and hairpins, which can affect the (3) ＿＿＿＿＿＿. And Mr. Bob need to practice (4) ＿＿＿＿＿＿ and put on special (5) ＿＿＿＿＿＿. Madelin will help Mr. Bob move from bed to (6) ＿＿＿＿＿＿.

✎ Notes

1. ward nurse 译为"病房护士"，其主要职责是认真执行各项护理制度和操作规程，正确执行医嘱，准确及时的完成各项护理工作等。

2. One more thing, the technician may ask you to take a deep breath and hold your breath while you having the CT scan.

还有一件事，当你进行 CT 扫描时，技师可能会要求你深呼吸并屏住呼吸。

hold your breath 译为"屏住呼吸"。

e. g. Hold your breath for a moment and exhale. 屏住呼吸片刻，然后呼气。

🎧 **Task 3　Listen to the conversation again and answer the following questions.**

听力 4.2

1. What procedure is Mr. Bob going to have?

＿＿

＿＿

2. What preparations should Mr. Bob make before performing CT examination?

＿＿

＿＿

3. How long does it going to take?

Notes

1. It is safe and painless. 它安全并且无痛。

"painless" 译为 "无痛"。 "less" 是后缀，表示 "无" 的意思， "fearless" 译为 "无畏的"，"childless" 译为 "无子女的"，"breathless" 译为 "无呼吸的"。

2. Transfer the intravenous fluid to the infusion rod of a wheelchair. 将静脉输液的液体转移到轮椅的输液杆上。

"intravenous fluid" 应译为 "输入静脉的液体"，intravenous 是指 "静脉内的"，"intra" 是前缀，表示 "在内"，"venous" 是词根，表示 "静脉的"，合成后表示静脉内的。静脉滴注可以用 "intravenous drip" 表示，静脉治疗可以用 "intravenous therapy" 来表示。

Task 4　**Put the following sentences from the conversation in the correct order. Listen again and check your answers.**

听力 4.2

Serial number	content
	You may stay in the radiology department for about an hour.
	I always wear wedding ring after I got married.
	Tomorrow I'll help you move from bed to wheelchair, and then transfer the intravenous fluid to the infusion rod of wheelchair.
	Thank you for your understanding and cooperation.
	Metal objects including jewelry, eyeglasses, dentures and hairpins may affect the CT images.
	The technician may ask you to take a deep breath and hold your breath while you having the CT scan.
	The CT examination has no pain and won't have a great impact on your body.
	I'll help you put on your special gown.
1	The doctor has ordered a chest CT examination according to your condition.
	I'll help you get ready before the porter comes.

Notes

1. We will take good care of it. 我们会把它保存好的。

take good care of 译为 "爱护，顾惜"

e. g. The nurses take good care of the patients. 护士对病人照应得很好。

Everybody has to take good care of the public property. 爱护公物，人人有责。

2. You may stay in the radiology department for about an hour. 您可能会在放射科停留大约一个小时。

"department" 在医学英语中一般译为 "科室"，可用 division、section 替代使用。如皮肤科，可以表达为 "department of dermatology" "division of dermatology" "section of dermaotolgy"。

Task 5 In pairs, practice taking a patient to Radiology for a CT. Student A, you are the nurse. Student B, you are the patient. Use the following prompts to help you. Swap roles and practice again.

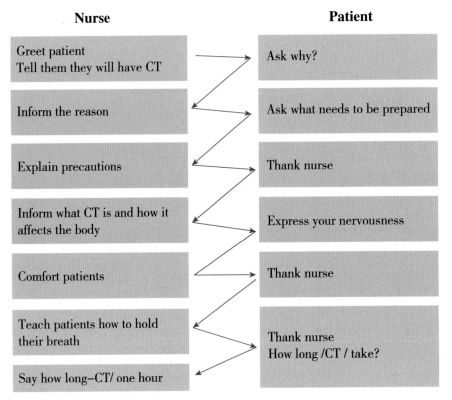

Nurse   **Patient**

Nurse	Patient
Greet patient Tell them they will have CT	Ask why?
Inform the reason	Ask what needs to be prepared
Explain precautions	Thank nurse
Inform what CT is and how it affects the body	Express your nervousness
Comfort patients	Thank nurse
Teach patients how to hold their breath	Thank nurse How long /CT / take?
Say how long–CT/ one hour	

Communication Tips:

Patient education needs to be comprehensive and easily understood. Nurse health educators must recognize that many patients lack their ability to understand health care information and what they need to do with that information. Here are some strategies the nurses can use to give instructions effectively.

1. Put the listeners at ease by using positive non – verbal communication such as hugging.

2. Sit or stand at the same level as the patient.

3. Use wording that's easy for your patients to understand.

4. Encourage by making remarks such as good job, well done, etc.

5. Engage patients by asking questions or having them repeat the instructions back to you.

Listening and Speaking

Activity 3　Preparing a Patient for Chest X – ray

Task 1　Match the terms (1 ~ 6) to their meanings (a ~ f).

1. Negative	a. To watch sb. /sth. carefully, especially to learn more about them.
2. Positive	b. The result of a test or an experiment which shows a substance or condition is present.
3. Oral	c. The result of a test or an experiment which shows a substance or condition is not present.

续表

4. Observe	d. Having an allergy to sth.
5. Allergic	e. Oral medicines are taken by mouth.
6. Rescue	f. To save sb. /sth. from a dangerous or harmful situation.

✖ Notes

Before imaging examination, patients should be prepared to understand the method, purpose and contraindications of imaging examination. In this process, some professional words will be involved, and their meanings need to be clear and understood accurately.

进行影像学检查之前需进行患者准备，让患者了解影像学检查的方法、目的以及有无禁忌证。在此过程中会涉及到一些专业词汇需明确其含义并准确理解。

Task 2　Listen to the conversation and circle the correct words.

Brandon, the Ward Nurse, is explaining the contents of the allergy test to Mr. Diego, a patient.　听力 4.3

1	Mr. Diego chose the **oral test / intradermal test** method.
2	Mr. Diego had a **penicillin / iodine** skin test before.
3	The intradermal test requires injection of **0. 1ml/1ml** iodine.
4	Observe the results **15 minutes / 20 minutes** after intravenous injection of contrast medium.
5	**Oral test / intradermal test** shall be conducted two days before contrast examination.

✖ Notes

1. Therefore, we need to do an allergy test before taking drugs. Only those who are negative can use them. 所以我们需要在服药前做一个过敏测试，只有结果为阴性的人才可以使用。

negative 本句中译为"阴性者，阴性的结果"。

false negatives 译为"假阴性"。临床工作中，有时存在假阴性的结果，故即使进行了过敏试验，在使用药物时也需进行严密观察、做好充分的抢救准备。

2. There are three main methods: oral test, intradermal test and intravenous injection. 主要有三种方法：口服试验、皮内试验和静脉注射。

oral 译为"口服的"。

e. g. It is oral medicine. 那是口服药。

3. Is it like penicillin skin test? 和青霉素皮试一样吗？

penicillin 译为"青霉素；盘尼西林"。

e. g. Penicillin cured him of pneumonia. 青霉素治好了他的肺炎。

听力 4.3

Task 3   Put the following sentences from the conversation in the correct order. Listen again and check your answers.

	Observe for 15 minutes to determine whether it is allergic.
	There are three main methods：oral test, intradermal test and intravenous injection.
	I have done a penicillin skin test.
	Just like penicillin skin test, inject it on the volar side of the forearm.
1	We need to do an allergy test before taking drugs, and only those who are negative can use them.
	Intradermal test is what we usually call skin test.

Notes

1. Injection was performed in the lower volar segment of the forearm.

在前臂掌侧下段进行注射。

lower volar segment of the forearm 译为"前臂掌侧下段"。

皮试常用部位为前臂掌侧下段，该部位皮肤薄、颜色浅、血管少，便于观察结果。

Task 4   Listen to the conversation and complete the following sentences.

听力 4.4

1. Mr. Diego will conduct _____ test now.

2. Let me _____ your skin with an antimicrobial swab.

3. Please be sure not to _____ or apply pressure to the injection site, ok?

4. A positive reaction to the test will cause a red, _____ , raised _____ .

Notes

1. intradermal test 译为"皮内注射"。

e. g. Conclusion：The safety of use of cephalosporins could be ensured by intradermal test. 结论：头孢菌素的皮试能确保其使用的安全性。

2. Will the shot hurt? 注射会疼吗？

"shot" 在医学英语中译为"注射"，当给患者注射时，可用"give a shot"表达。

e. g. The vaccine is given by shots to provide immunization against diseases. 可以通过注射疫苗提供对疾病的免疫。

Task 5   Work in pairs and practice doing an allergy test with each other. Student A, you are the nurse；Student B, you are the patient. Use the information below to help you. Swap roles and practice again.

Intradermal injection（Allergy test）	
Purpose	The main purpose is to determine whether the patient is allergic to a drug.
Injection site	Lower volar segment of forearm.
Injection dose	0. 1ml
Result judgment	A positive reaction to the test will cause a red, itchy, raised bump, with a diameter of more than 1cm.
Points for attention	Do not massage or press the injection site, and try not to leave the ward within 20 minutes.

Communication Tips:

Communication barriers often go undetected in health care settings and can have serious effects on the health and safety of patients. Promoting patient comprehension of health care recommendations is essential to the effective delivery of health care. The nurses may use some expressions to check understanding.

1. Could you repeat back the steps for me so I can be sure you followed my explanation?
2. Do you see what I mean?
3. Could you tell me what step one is?
4. Can you show me how you'll inject insulin at home?

Writing

With wide use of X-rays in physical examinations, people are increasingly concerned about exposure to radiation. Please express your opinion, which should include: ①Whether you agree to the imaging examination; ②The important role of imaging examination; ③If too much imaging is dangerous; ④Can it lead to cancer or other complications?

Proverbs and Sayings

✧ Active listening is generally a more effective communication tool than passive listening. 主动倾听一般来说是一种比被动倾听更有效的工具。

✧ Appropriate humor is an integral part of communication.
适当的幽默是交流的必要构成部分。

✧ Conflict resolution is best achieved through using a courteous yet assertive approach, instead of resorting to passivity or aggression.
解决冲突的最好态度是礼貌且自信而不是被动或夹击。

书网融合……

听力材料4.1　　　　听力材料4.2　　　　听力材料4.3　　　　听力材料4.4

Unit 5　Caring for Operative Patients

PPT

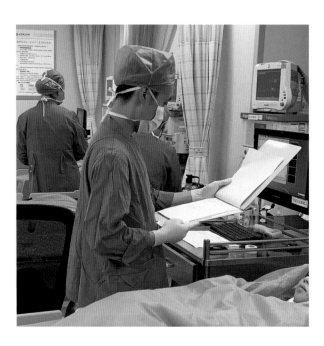

Reading part:

Be familiar with the steps and significance of the perioperative management of ERAS.

Listening and Speaking part:

1. Be able to do preoperative visits and fill out the preoperative visit sheet.

2. Be able to paraphrase medical words and answer patient's questions smoothly.

3. Be able to relieve the patient's anxiety.

4. Be able to make preoperative requirements clearly and accurately.

5. Be able to perform tripartite verification in the operating room.

6. Be able to know the indicators that need to be tested during the post – anesthesia recovery room.

Writing part:

Be able to write a preoperative check report which is clinical and factual, using appropriate medical terminology, accurate grammar and punctuation.

Warm – up Exercises

Elva is a nurse who is responsible for preparing operation in the operation room. Can you help her to label the items and explain the function?

> Indwelling urinary catheter;   Drainage catheter;   Antibiotics;
>
> Endotracheal cannula;   Patient Controlled Analgesic (PCA) pump;
>
> Ventilator;   Monitor;   Surgical incision dressing;   Intravenous indwelling needle

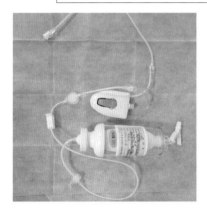

A

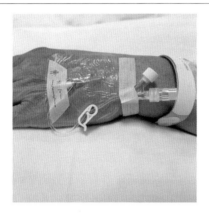

B

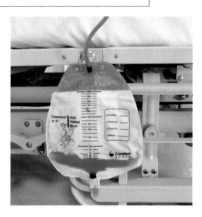

C

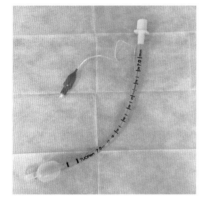

D

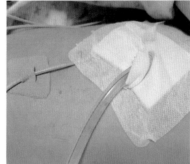

E

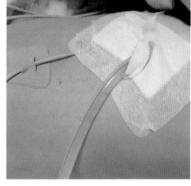

F

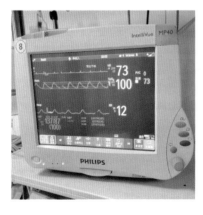

G

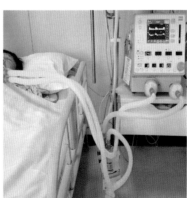

H

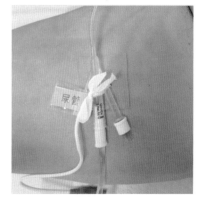

I

Reading

The Perioperative Management of ERAS

ERAS aims to reduce trauma and stress, maintain a stable environment in the body, ensure normal physiological functions of the body, and promote patient recovery. Enhanced recovery nursing is on the basis of evidence-based nursing, based on holistic nursing, and taking nursing intervention as measures to optimize and integrate the latest nursing concepts, establish clinical nursing procedures, implement clinical nursing pathways, and achieve the purpose of accelerating rehabilitation.

Preoperative preparation

Preoperative preparation includes preoperative education, nutrition screening, preventive application of antibacterial drugs and antithrombotic therapy, individualized blood pressure and blood sugar control and corresponding management plans.

(1) Preoperative education

Health education can be carried out through oral, written or multimedia forms. The content includes detailed introduction of the ward environment, supervisory doctors, nurses, hospitals and wards related rules and regulations; detailed knowledge of preoperative care and various concepts to promote recovery to relieve patient's tension, anxiety, and fear.

(2) Screening and treatment of malnutrition

Nutritional risk screening (NRS2002) is recommended as the preferred tool for nutritional risk screening after admission. Nutritional risk score ≥3 points indicates that the patient has nutritional risk. Oral nutrition or enteral nutrition is the preferred method of preoperative nutritional support.

(3) Fasting and oral carbohydrates

The primary nurse instructs patients without gastrointestinal motility disorders to fast 6 hours from solid diet and 2 hours from clear liquids before the operation. The patient without history of diabetes should drink 400ml of a 12.5% carbohydrate beverage 2 hours before surgery, which can reduce the incidence of postoperative insulin resistance and hyperglycemia and relieve hunger, thirst, and anxiety.

(4) Preventive antithrombotic treatment

It is recommended to use the Caprini risk assessment scale for risk assessment of VTE. It is should take basic prevention, mechanical prevention, and drug prevention measures according to the patient's thrombosis risk stratification.

(5) Pulmonary rehabilitation exercise

Instruct patients to quit smoking before surgery (at least 2 weeks), and to perform effective coughing, postural drainage, chest and back flapping, which help patients maintain airway smoothness and clear respiratory secretions in time.

(6) Other

Primary nurses should complete bowel preparation, skin preparation, partial preparation of certain surgical specialties, blood preparation, allergy test, preventive application of antibacterial drugs and preoperative sedative medications according to doctor's orders.

Surgery day

The primary nurse and the operating room personnel carefully check the patient's identity and information, and do the handover work of preoperative and postoperative. Before the operation, the surgeon, anesthesiologist, and operating room nurse should conduct a tripartite check on the patient. During the operation, the operating room nurse should control the patient's fluid intake, and keep the patient's central body temperature more than 36℃. The patient's situation should be communicated and fed back among the ward, the operating room, and the anesthesia recovery room in time.

Post – operative care

After returning to the ward, the primary nurse closely observes the patient's vital signs and condition changes, and follows the doctor's instructions to use drugs such as acid suppression, antiemetic, anti – inflammatory, hemostasis, analgesia, nutrition, etc. Meanwhile, the nurse should implement intervention measures of ERAS nursing: early post – op feeding, early ambulation, drainage tube care, breathing exercises, etc.

(522 words)

✂ Notes

1. ERAS aims to reduce trauma and stress, maintain a stable environment in the body, ensure normal physiological functions of the body, and promote patient recovery.

本句中"ERAS"全写为"Enhanced Recovery after Surgery",意为加速康复外科,是指通过应用基于循证证据的围术期处理措施,达到减少术后并发症、提高手术安全性、加速康复的目的。

ERAS 已迅速成为 21 世纪一项重要的外科学进展与革命。ERAS 是由多学科共同协作,其中加速康复外科护理是重点内容,是以循证护理为依据的个性化康复护理。

2. Nutritional risk screening 经常缩写为 NRS2002,意为营养风险筛查,是由医护人员实施的简便的筛查方法,用以决定是否需要制定或实施肠外肠内营养支持计划,是欧洲肠外肠内营养学会(ESPEN)于 2002 年推荐使用的筛查工具。目前该工具是可以用于我国的比较好的营养风险筛查工具。

3. Fasting and oral carbohydrates

"fast"在本文中意为"禁食",其也有我们熟知的"快的,快速地"含义。

e. g. All patients were fasted before surgery.

所有的病人在做外科手术前都不能吃东西。

"oral"本文中意为"口服",口服有多种表达方法,如"taken orally, Per Os, PO",比如:antibiotic tablets taken orally,口服抗生素片。

4. "Primary nurse"意为"责任护士",不要译为"主要护士"或者"初级护士"。

5. VTE:Venous Thrombus Embolism,静脉血栓栓塞症。

6. Caprini risk assessment scale,Caprini 风险评估量表

Caprini 风险评估量表是一种有效、简单方便的 VTE 风险预测评估工具;能有效帮助临床医生鉴别 VTE 高危患者,辅助预防方案的选择,从而减少 VTE 发生率。该表包含了大约 40 个不同的血栓形成危险因素,基本涵盖了外科手术和住院患者可能发生 VTE 的所有危险因素,通过这些因素对患者进行 VTE 风险评分。

After – reading Exercises

Task 1   Match the words with their proper meaning.

1. Holistic	a. 抗菌药、抗生素
2. Preoperative	b. 营养失调、营养不良
3. Antibacterial	c. 术后的
4. Antithrombotic	d. 抗血栓的
5. Ward	e. 整体的
6. Malnutrition	f. 肺部的
7. Carbohydrate	g. 术前的
8. Postoperative	h. 麻醉师、麻醉医生
9. Pulmonary	i. 碳水化合物
10. Anesthesiologist	j. 病房

Task 2   Think about the following questions and write down your answer.

1. What is enhanced recovery nursing?

_____

_____

2. Write down the steps a nurse should follow about perioperative management of ERAS.

Ⅰ. Preoperative Preparation

_____

_____

Ⅱ. Surgery Day

_____

_____

Ⅲ. Post – operative Care

_____

_____

Task 3   Complete the following sentences with a word or short phrase from the text.

1. Preoperative preparation includes _____, nutrition screening, preventive application of _____ and antithrombotic therapy, individualized _____ and _____ and corresponding management plans.

2. The primary nurse instructs patients to fast _____ hours from solid diet and _____ hours from clear liquids before the operation.

3. The patient without history of diabetes should drink _____ ml of a _____% carbohydrate beverage _____ hours before surgery.

4. Before the operation, _____, _____, and _____ should conduct a tripartite check on the patient.

Listening and Speaking

Activity 1   Doing a Preoperative Check

Task 1   Match the following medical terms (1 ~ 10) with paraphrases (a ~ j).

1. Arthroplasty	a. a drug that reduces excitability and calms a person
2. Occurrence	b. urine output
3. Gastrointestinal tract	c. a drug that reduces high blood pressure
4. Gastric contents reflux	d. a disease of frequent occurrence
5. Aspiration	e. replacement of a malformed or degenerated joint
6. Anti – hypertensive drug	f. tubular passage of mucous membrane and muscle extending about 8. 3 meters from mouth to anus
7. Sedative drug	g. the passages through which air enters and leaves the body
8. Hypnotic drug	h. a drug that induces sleep
9. UOP	i. the act of inhaling
10. Respiratory tract	j. backflow of stomach contents

Notes

Perfect preoperative preparation can make patients have sufficient psychological preparation and good physiological conditions. If nurses find that patients may have conditions affect the operation, such as changes in patients' condition, menstruation of women, fasting not according to the doctor's instructions, etc. , they should report to the doctor in time. If the patients are not suitable for the operation, the operation should be delayed or canceled if necessary.

完善的术前准备可使患者具有充分的心理准备和良好的生理条件，护理人员若发现患者有可能影响手术的情况，例如：患者病情变化、女性月经来潮、未按医嘱禁食等，应及时报告医师，经评估不宜实施手术者，必要时延迟或取消手术。

Task 2   Listen to the conversation 5. 1 between Sarah, the Ward Nurse, and Mr. Steward, the patient. Mark the following options True (T) or False (F).

听力 5. 1

( ) 1. Mr. Steward did not agree with smoking cessation for operation.

( ) 2. Sarah didn't give a detailed explanation on necessity of smoking cessation.

( ) 3. The nurse asked Mr. Steward to fast 10 hours from solid diet and 4 hours from water before the operation, and explained it.

( ) 4. Mr. Steward's surgery requires skin preparation.

( ) 5. Mr. Steward has a sleep disorder.

( ) 6. Sarah did not ask Mr. Steward to remove the jewelry before entering the operating room.

✂ Notes

1. Lung infections 是指肺部感染，戒烟4周可降低围手术期并发症发生率。

2. Deep breathing 深呼吸，effective cough 有效咳嗽，均是预防肺部感染的重要措施。

3. Gastric contents reflux and aspiration 是指胃内容物返流及误吸，麻醉药物会使全身肌肉松弛，胃贲门括约肌扩张，此时胃内容物易返流至咽喉腔内，同时由于咽喉反射减弱，胃内容物进入气道会造成误吸。

Task 3 **Listen to the conversation again, and write the right options in the right column.**

听力 5.1

Terms	Corresponding options
1. Total knee arthroplasty	_____
2. Indwelling urinary Catheter	_____
3. Respiratory tract preparation	_____
4. Gastrointestinal tract preparation	_____
5. Hypertension	_____

a. Quit smoking and take deep breathing and effective sputum excretion exercises

b. Fasted 6～8 hours from solid diet and 2 hours from clear liquids to prevent suffocation or aspiration pneumonia due to anesthesia or vomiting caused by surgery.

c. To inset a catheter into bladder

d. Operation of knee replacement

e. High blood pressure

✂ Notes

Indwelling urinary catheter 是指留置导尿，术前留置导尿的主要目的是术中可通过观察尿量及时了解肾功能，决定输液速度、输液量，并且术后可防止尿潴留。术后应尽早拔除导尿管，以降低泌尿系统感染风险。

Task 4 **Listen to the conversation again and complete the following sentences with a word or short phrase.**

听力 5.1

1. Mr. Steward is scheduled to have _____ _____ _____ _____ _____ at _____ tomorrow.

2. Don't worry. I will help to _____ _____ _____ before the operation. I hope you can _____ _____ the operation _____ .

3. Respiratory tract preparation means _____ smoking and do some respiratory exercises, such as _____ _____ _____ and _____ _____ training.

4. _____ tract preparation is mainly to prevent _____ _____ _____ and _____ after anesthesia.

5. Tomorrow morning, please put on the _____ _____ . Remove your _____ , _____ and _____ before operation. Leave your _____ and mobile phone to your family for safekeeping.

Notes

easy – to – understand language 是指通俗易懂的语言，在与术前患者沟通时，尽量避免生涩难懂的医学术语，同时可配合使用图片、视频等材料进行辅助讲解。

Task 5　In pairs，play the roles of nurse and patient，using the 5.1 conversation script.

Nurse	Patient
Do the self-introduction	Ask the nurse what is the purpose of the operation
Explain the operation	Tell the nurse his feeling
Relieve the patient	Say thank you
Ask the patient about quitting smoking	Answer the question
Tell the patient that he should do respiratory tract preparation	Ask the nurse what is meaning of respiratory tract preparation
Tell the patient how to do respiratory tract preparation	Say okay
Tell the patient how to do gastrointestinal tract preparation	Say okay
Ask the patient the medical history: hypertension, or high blood pressure	Answer that he has high blood pressure and ask whether to take drugs as usual
Tell the patient that a nurse will take the blood pressure and then make a decision by the doctor	Say okay
Tell the patient to take a bath	Say okay and tell nurse he couldn't sleep well
Tell the patient that the doctor will prescribe drugs for him	Say thank you
Tell the patient to put on patient's grown, remove stuff	Say yes
Tell the patient what to do in the operation room and after the operation	Say okay

👤 Communication Tips：

In communicating with patients, nurses should try their best to embody humanistic care and patiently answer questions raised by patients, so as to alleviate or eliminate patients' doubts and fears.

e. g.

1. Good morning/afternoon, Mrs. / Mr. X, do you know you're scheduled to have an operation tomorrow？

2. I would like to explain the preparation for the operation. If you have any question, please stop and tell me.

3. You look worried. Do you have any problems？

4. Don't worry. It's a common operation.

5. You are going to have general anesthesia. During the operation you'll feel nothing.

6. You'll find yourself back in your room after the operation.

Listening and Speaking

Activity 2　Filling a Preoperative Checklist

🎧 **Task 1　Listen to the conversation 5. 2 between Elva and Mr. Steward, and match the words or phrases with the explanations on the right.**

听力 5. 2

Elva, a theatre nurse, is giving the preoperative education to Mr. Steward.

1. Preoperative visit	a. The movement of arms and legs
2. Orthopedics	b. The theatre nurses visit the patients in the ward before the operation.
3. Osteoarthritis	c. A surgical specialty which treat diseases or injuries to the skeletal system.
4. Arthroplasty	d. A progressive, degenerative joint disease, the most common form of arthritis, especially in older persons.
5. Limbs moving	e. Surgical reconstruction of a joint to relieve pain or restore motion.
6. Knee joints	f. Joint connection of thigh and lower leg.

✂ Notes

The theatre nurses will visit the patients in the ward before the operation, learn about the patients' basic situation and allergy history, etc. , and introduce the operating room environment and procedures to patients and their families, and explain precautions.

手术室护士会在手术前到病房访视患者，了解患者的基本情况和过敏史等，向患者及其家属介绍手术室环境及流程，并交代注意事项。

Task 2　Listen to the conversation 5. 2，and fill in the operation patient visit record sheet.

听力 5. 2

General condition of the patient	
Hospital number：＿＿＿＿　Bed number：＿＿＿＿ Name：＿＿＿＿＿＿＿　Age：＿＿＿＿＿ Gender：＿＿＿＿＿＿＿ Department：＿＿＿＿＿＿＿	Preoperative diagnosis：＿＿＿＿＿＿＿ Name of proposed operation：＿＿＿＿＿＿ ＿＿＿＿＿＿＿＿＿＿＿＿＿＿＿＿＿ Planned operation time：＿＿＿＿＿＿＿

Operation history：Yes（　）　　No（　）

Past history：＿＿＿＿＿＿＿＿＿＿＿＿＿

Allergy history：No（　）　　Yes（　）

Blood type：A（　）　B（　）　AB（　）　O（　）　RH（　+　　−）

Blood－borne diseases：No（　）　Yes（　）

Vein condition：Filled（　）　generally hard（　）　not touchable（　）

Physical activity：free（　）　obstacles（　）

Skin condition：intact（　）　damaged：＿＿＿＿＿

Nutritional status：good（　）　average（　）　poor（　）

Notes

1. Blood type 是指血型，常用的血型系统包括 ABO 血型系统和 Rh 血型系统，前者包括 A 型、B 型、AB 型和 O 型，后者包括 Rh 阴性和 Rh 阳性。

2. Blood－borne diseases 是指血液传播疾病，是一类经血液、体液途径传播的传染性疾病，常见的有乙型肝炎，丙型肝炎，梅毒以及艾滋病。

Task 3　Listen to the conversation 5. 3 and answer the following questions.

听力 5. 3

1. What are the vital signs the nurse measured?

＿＿＿＿＿＿＿＿＿＿＿＿＿＿＿＿＿＿＿＿＿＿＿＿＿＿＿＿＿＿＿＿＿＿＿＿＿＿＿

＿＿＿＿＿＿＿＿＿＿＿＿＿＿＿＿＿＿＿＿＿＿＿＿＿＿＿＿＿＿＿＿＿＿＿＿＿＿＿

2. When did the patient take last food and water?

＿＿＿＿＿＿＿＿＿＿＿＿＿＿＿＿＿＿＿＿＿＿＿＿＿＿＿＿＿＿＿＿＿＿＿＿＿＿＿

＿＿＿＿＿＿＿＿＿＿＿＿＿＿＿＿＿＿＿＿＿＿＿＿＿＿＿＿＿＿＿＿＿＿＿＿＿＿＿

3. Which part did the nurse check before operation?

＿＿＿＿＿＿＿＿＿＿＿＿＿＿＿＿＿＿＿＿＿＿＿＿＿＿＿＿＿＿＿＿＿＿＿＿＿＿＿

＿＿＿＿＿＿＿＿＿＿＿＿＿＿＿＿＿＿＿＿＿＿＿＿＿＿＿＿＿＿＿＿＿＿＿＿＿＿＿

Notes

The ward nurses conduct the preoperative nursing evaluation again on the day of the operation. The contents of the preoperative evaluation are consistent with the contents of the preoperative health education and the "surgical patient handover form", so as to confirm the patient's identity information and all the preoperative preparations, and the operation can be carried out according to the original plan.

病房护士在患者手术当日再次进行术前护理评估，术前评估内容与患者术前健康宣教以及《手术患者交接单》上的内容一致，以确认患者身份信息及所有术前准备就绪，可以按原计划手术。

听力 5.4

Task 4 Listen to the conversation 5. 4 and choose the items the operation requires. (   )

A. Medical records

B. Four imaging films

C. Two antibiotics ceftriaxone

D. Surgical hemostasis sponge

E. Fixation band

F. One 0. 9% saline solution 100ml

Notes

The "surgical patient handover form" is filled in by the ward nurses, and the contents include the patient's status and items. The patient's status includes the patient's identity confirmation, vital signs, the time of the last intake, whether there are removable dentures, jewelry, glasses, etc., whether the female is in the menstrual period, infusion channel, indwelling pipeline, skin condition, etc., and the items include medical records, images, medication type and quantity, other items, etc. After filling in the form, nurses and operating room staff signed for confirmation.

《手术患者交接单》由病房护士填写，填写内容包括患者情况及所带物品，患者情况包括患者身份确认、生命体征、最后一次进食进水时间、是否有活动义齿、首饰、眼镜等、女性是否在月经期、输液通道、留置管路情况、皮肤情况等，所带物品包括病历、影像片、药品名称及数量、其他物品情况等。填写完后病房护士和手术室人员签字确认。

Task 5 In pairs, according to the information below, practise the conversation between the ward nurse and the patient on the day of operation.

Surgical Patient Handover Form	
Patient status	Identity/bracelet confirmation：Yes√ No T 36. 7℃ P 78 time/minute R 18 time/minute Bp 135/84 mmHg Weight 84. 5kg Last drinking time：18：00 on Aug 16th, 2021 Last Eating time：5：30 on Aug 17th, 2021 Movable dentures, jewelry, glasses：No√ Yes Female during menstruation：Yes No√ Surgery site identification：Yes√ No Infusion：Yes√ Location：the back of the left hand No Pipeline：Yes Name：_____ No√ Skin：Normal√ Abnormal High risk of pressure ulcers：Yes No√ Other：No
Items	☑Medical Records ☑Imaging films：__4__ （quantity） Drug：No Yes√ Drug name and quantity：Two antibiotics ceftriaxone, and one 0. 9% saline solution 100ml. Item：No√ Yes Item name and quantity：_____
Signature of handover/receiving personnel：	
Handover time：	

Communication Tips：

For special issues related to the surgical process or prognosis, try to keep with the tone of the surgeon as consistent as possible, avoid detailed explanations, and ask the doctor in charge to explain if necessary, so as to avoid adverse consequences or medical disputes.

E. g. ：

1. Did your doctor tell what sort of operation you are going to have?

2. It's hard to tell. It will depend on operating procedure and your recovery from the anesthesia.

3. I'm sorry I can't say, it will depend on our investigations and the doctor's diagnosis.

Listening and Speaking

Activity 3   Caring for a Patient in Recovery Room

Task 1   In pairs, complete the sentences using the words and phrases on the right.

1. If patients have severe heart problems, they go to ...	a. PACU (Post Anaesthesia Care Unit)
2. If patients are too ill to go to the ward, they go to ...	b. ICU (Intensive Care Unit)
3. ... is where patients go to wake up after general anesthesia with tracheal intubation.	c. Ward
4. If patients are alert and oriented and their vital signs are normal after operation, they go to ...	d. CCU (Coronary Care Unit)

Notes

PACU (Post Anaesthesia Care Unit), also known as post – anaesthesia monitoring treatment room, refers to a ward that monitors and treats patients after anesthesia and surgery, so that patients can survive the anesthesia recovery period and stabilize their vital signs.

麻醉恢复室，又称麻醉后监测治疗室，指对麻醉及手术后患者进行监测和治疗，使患者平稳度过麻醉恢复期及生命体征恢复稳定的病室。

Task 2   Listen to the conversation 5.5, mark the items that Mr. Steward needs to be monitored with a "√".

听力 5.5

Mr. Steward has been completed the operation and was transferred to the anesthesia recovery room to wait for recovery and extubation. Elva, the theatre nurse, Calvin, is the recovery nurse. Elva hands Mr. Steward to Calvin.

□body temperature	□surgical incision dressing
□blood pressure	□the fixation and drainage of the patient's drainage tube
□respiratory rate and tidal volume	□thirsty
□consciousness	□IV infusion

✂ Notes

Tidal volume means the volume of air inspired or expired during each normal, quiet respiratory cycle. Common abbreviations are TV or V with subscript T.

潮气量是指每个正常的平静呼吸周期吸入或呼出的气量。常缩写为 TV 或带脚注 T 的 V（V_T）。机械通气的病人需要关注潮气量的变化。

Adult tidal volume is equal to kilogram body weight multiply by 6~8ml. Tidal volume is too large or too small will affect patients. Excessive tidal volume will cause excessive alveolar expansion and excessive ventilation, leading to ventilator related lung injury. Tidal volume is too small will cause alveolar collapse, blood oxygen decline, carbon dioxide retention, leading to organ dysfunction.

成人潮气量等于千克体重乘以 6~8ml，潮气量过大或过小都会对患者造成影响，潮气量过大，肺泡过度膨胀，会造成过度通气，导致呼吸机相关性肺损伤，潮气量过小，肺泡萎陷，血氧下降，二氧化碳潴留，引起各器官功能不全。

🎧 **Task 3 Listen to the conversation 5.6, and write down the procedure of judging the patient's consciousness is restored or not after general anesthesia with tracheal intubation.**

听力 5.6

1. _____

2. _____

3. _____

✂ Notes

There are many different assessment tools for neurological function. However, the most widely used tool is the Glasgow Coma Scale (GCS). The GCS includes three areas of neurological function: Eye – opening（睁眼反应），Verbal response（语言反应），Motor response（肢体运动）.

Eye – opening	
Spontaneous 自主睁眼	4
To sound 呼唤睁眼	3
To Pain 刺痛睁眼	2
No eye – opening 无反应	1
Verbal response	
Oriented 回答正确	5
Confused 回答错乱	4
Inappropriate words 答非所问	3
Incomprehensible sounds 只能发声	2
No verbal response 无反应	1

（续表）

Motor response	
Obeys commands 遵嘱运动	6
Localizing response to pain 刺痛定位	5
Withdrawal response to pain 刺痛躲避	4
Flexion to pain 刺痛过屈	3
Extension to pain 刺痛过伸	2
No motor response 无反应	1

The GCS is scored between 3 and 15, 3 being the worst and 15 the best. A score of 13 or higher correlates with mild consciousness disorder, a score of 9 to 12 correlates with moderate consciousness disorder, and a score of 8 or less represents severe consciousness disorder.

Task 4　Listen to the conversation 5. 6, and sort the steps to remove the tracheal intubation tube in the correct order.

听力 5. 6

1. _____　2. _____　3. _____　4. _____　5. _____

A. Empty Airbag

B. Oxygen inhalation

C. Suction

D. Remove the fixture that secures the tracheal intubation tube

E. Cooperate with spontaneous coughing while extubating the tube

Notes

1. Tracheal intubation tube 是指气管内插管。

2. Extubation of endotracheal tube 是指拔除气管内插管。

intubate 和 extubate 是一对反义词，前者指插管，后者指拔管。

Task 5　In pairs, describe the procedures how to evaluate patients in the anesthesia recovery room to your partner.

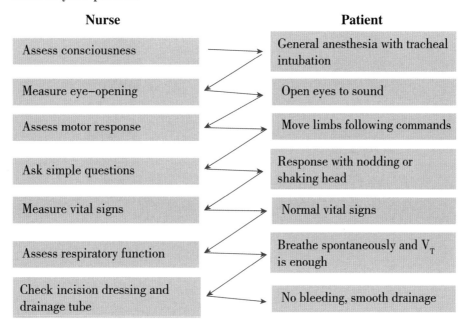

Nurse	Patient
Assess consciousness	General anesthesia with tracheal intubation
Measure eye-opening	Open eyes to sound
Assess motor response	Move limbs following commands
Ask simple questions	Response with nodding or shaking head
Measure vital signs	Normal vital signs
Assess respiratory function	Breathe spontaneously and V_T is enough
Check incision dressing and drainage tube	No bleeding, smooth drainage

Communication Tips：

When giving health education to patients with general anesthesia through oral endotracheal intubation, nurses should use reassuring voices and intonations. Nurses should explain the situations to patients using simplified, clear and relevant language. For example：

1. If you can hear us, please open eyes, shake hands or raise legs.

2. When you are fully awake and your condition is stable, we will have professional medical staff to escort you to the ward.

Writing

If you are Nurse Sarah, please write a short report about preoperative checks before the operation. It should include patient's information, vital signs, last food and water intake time, infusion channel, indwelling pipeline, surgical site, etc.

Proverbs and Sayings

✧ I hold patients' hands during the scariest flight of their lives.

在病人最恐惧不安的时刻，我就在他们身边，紧握着他们的双手。

✧ Leave the bitterness, tiredness and resentment to yourself, and give happiness, safety and health to the patient.

把苦、累、怨留给自己，把乐、安、康送给病人。

✧ The patient is in my heart, the recovery is in my hand.

病人在我心中，康复在我手中。

书网融合……

听力材料5.1　　听力材料5.2　　听力材料5.3

听力材料5.4　　听力材料5.5　　听力材料5.6

Unit 6　Discharging Patients

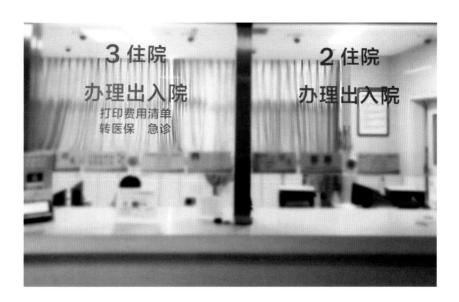

Learning Objectives

Reading part：

Be able to identify the details of discharge instruction.

Listening and Speaking part：

1. Be able to identify and recognize specific information on discharge instructions for patients.

2. Be able to perform discharge education effectively for patients.

3. Be able to correctly explain discharge summary and discharge plan to patients, using effective communication strategies and building a good nurse-patient relationship.

4. Be able to know the necessary information about referral of discharged patients to other medical structures.

5. Be able to use effective communication strategies to improve the nurse-patient relationship.

Writing part：

Be able to write a patient referral letter, using appropriate medical terminology, accurate grammar and punctuation.

Warm-up Exercises

Eliza is a nurse who is giving some discharge instructions to a patient. Match the pictures with these items.

Diet	Medication	Sports and exercise
Living habits	Recheck	Discharge summary

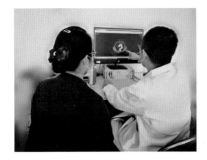

A _____

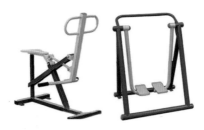

B _____

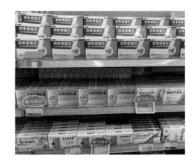

C _____

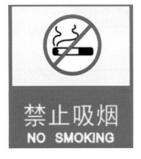

D _____

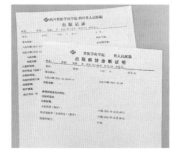

E _____

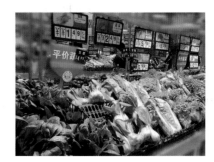

F _____

Reading

阅读译文

Discharge Instructions for Patients: Best Practices

Hospital discharge is cited as a vulnerable point in a patient's care transition. Its effective execution has significant implications on a patient's recovery trajectory. The most effective tool in a clinician's toolbox to promote patient healing is the effective delivery of communicating discharge instructions for patients.

Best Practices

A successfully planned and executed hospital discharge is critically important to a patient's continued recovery and fulfillment of post-discharge care. The discharge conversation initiated by both the attending clinician and the discharging nurse must contain all pertinent information necessary to ensure a safe departure from the hospital and successful follow-up.

It is also important to have a family member, friend, caretaker or home health aide engaged in the conversation. The following are some of the important points that should be discussed:

◇ Patients must understand the medical or surgical reasons for their current admission and what transpired during the hospitalization.

◇ Patients must have a clear understanding of their medical conditions and what must be done to continue care as an outpatient.

◇ Patients must receive an explanation of potential warning signs and symptoms that could arise.

◇ Patients should be provided with a 24-hour phone number for emergencies.

◇ Patients should have the name of the provider responsible for their care after discharge (provide written name, address and phone number).

Provide Clear Discharge Instructions

All instructions for care at home, including medications, diet, therapy, and follow-up appointments, must be explained in detail to all patients and then presented in written form to take home upon discharge.

Exact dates and times of follow-up appointments need to be included. Providers must inform patients of any pending lab work or tests that need to be checked, and of course, ensure they have transportation at the time of discharge.

A written list with all medications must be explained in detail and presented to patients. Patients need to fully understand when and how to take their medications. Providers must explain potential side effects and associated warnings concerning the medications.

Summary

The importance of communicating clear discharge instructions to patients cannot be understated.

As a significant number of patients discharged from the hospital return within 14~30 days, discharge discussions must confirm that patients understand their medical conditions and all information required for a successful post-discharge period, including medications and follow-up appointments.

(398 words)

✂ Notes

1. The most effective tool in a clinician's toolbox to promote patient healing is the effective delivery of communicating discharge instructions for patients.

在临床医生的工具箱中，促进患者康复的最有效工具是为患者提供有效的出院指导信息。

本句中"heal"意为"治疗，康复"，侧重指治愈伤口，多指创伤，外伤等。其它表示"治疗"之意的词还有：①cure：侧重指治愈内部疾病；②treat：侧重指用药物、手术等治疗疾病或创伤，不涉及治愈的结果。

e. g. This medicine will promote the healing of the wound.

这种药物会促进伤口的愈合。

2. A successfully planned and executed hospital discharge is critically important to a patient's continued recovery and fulfillment of post-discharge care.

成功地计划并完成出院对于患者的持续康复和完成出院后的护理至关重要。

本句中"post-discharge"翻译为"出院后"，"post-"为前缀，来源于拉丁语，意为"after, behind"，表示"在后面"。

e. g. Post-discharge follow-up without pain recurrence. 出院后随访无疼痛再发。

3. to ensure a safe departure from the hospital and successful follow-up.

以确保安全出院并成功进行随访。

本句中"follow-up"不是"后续行动，后续事物"的意思，而是应翻译为"定期复查，随访"，是医院对出院的患者以通讯或其他方式，定期了解患者病情变化和指导患者康复的一种观察方法。

e. g. The patient was seen for follow-up visits once every two months.

这位病人每两个月接受一次随访就诊。

4. Patients should have the name of the provider responsible for their care after discharge.

患者应被告知出院后负责照护他们的医疗机构信息。

本句中"provider"意为"healthcare provider"是指医疗服务的提供者，本句中可译为"医疗机构"。

e. g. If your child has a fever for 3 or more days with 2 or 3 of these classic symptoms, you should bring your child to the doctor or other healthcare provider.

如果您的孩子出现3天以上的发热，并伴有2~3个典型的症状，应该带您的孩子去看医生或其他医务工作人员。

After – reading Exercises

Task 1　Match the words with their proper meaning.

1. recovery trajectory	a. 护理人员
2. discharge instruction	b. 护理过渡
3. follow-up	c. 出院后护理
4. post-discharge care	d. 康复轨迹
5. care transition	e. 出院指导
6. home health aide	f. 潜在副作用
7. medical condition	g. 医疗状况
8. promote patient healing	h. 家庭保健助手
9. potential side effects	i. 随访
10. caretaker	j. 促进患者康复

Task 2　Complete the following sentences with a word or short phrase from the text.

1. ＿＿＿＿＿＿＿＿ is considered to be a weak link in the transition of patient care.

2. The discharge conversation initiated by the attending clinician and ＿＿＿＿＿＿＿ must contain all necessary relevant information.

3. When the patient is discharged, all home care instructions, including medications, diet, therapy, and ＿＿＿＿＿＿＿, must be explained to the patient.

4. ＿＿＿＿＿＿＿ must inform patients of any laboratory work or tests that need to be examined.

5. According to the passage, a large number of discharged patients will return to the hospital within ＿＿＿＿＿＿＿.

Task 3　In pairs, discuss the following questions.

1. What are the key points to achieve best practices in discharging patients?

_____

_____

_____

2. What instructions should be provided to patients when they are discharged?

_____

_____

_____

Listening and Speaking

Activity 1　Giving Instructions to Patients – 1 (Diet and Medication)

Task 1　The following are some of the contents that must be included in the discharge summary. Work in pairs, match these contents (1 ~ 10) with their Chinese meaning (a ~ j).

Discharge Summary	
1.　Discharge Instructions	a.　主治医生
2.　Attending Diagnosis	b.　出院日期
3.　Discharge Medications	c.　病历号
4.　Hospital Course	d.　病人姓名
5.　Attending Physician	e.　出院诊断
6.　Medical Record Number	f.　入院日期
7.　Discharge Diagnosis	g.　出院药物
8.　Discharge Date	h.　入院诊断
9.　Admission Date	i.　出院说明
10.　Patient Name	j.　住院诊治经过

✎ Notes

Discharge summary is a clinical report prepared by health professionals at the end of hospitalization or a series of treatment. It is a summary of the diagnosis and treatment of patients in hospital. It is not only the main way of communication between the hospital care team and the aftercare provider, but also convenient for future follow-up visit as a reference.

出院小结是由医疗专业人员在住院或一系列治疗结束时编写的临床报告，是对住院病人的诊断和治疗的总结。它不仅是医院护理团队和后续护理医疗机构之间的主要沟通方式，也便于以后复诊时作为参考。

Task 2 In pairs, discuss the discharge summary below and point out what the letters "A ~ F" stand for.

Discharge Summary

A : *Benjamin Englhart*

Medical Record Number：100254689

Admission Date：29/06/2019

B : *15/07/2019*

C : *Dr. Gary Marshall*

Attending Diagnosis：*RLL pneumonia, COPD exacerbation*

D *L pneumonia, COPD exacerbation, mild CHF*

E : *72 years old thin white male presented to emergency on 06/29/2019 with shortness of breath, weakness and dehydration. Chest X-ray showed right lower lobe infiltrate, ABGs unremarkable.*

1) Pneumonia：treated with ceftriaxone and azithromycin iv. Switched to PO after 72 hours.

2) Exacerbation of COPD：patient treated with inhaled and oral steroids.

3) Weakness and dehydration：secondary to pneumonia and COPD. Responded well to strengthening with PT and regular meals.

Discharge Medications：*Azithromycin daily until gone*

F : *no activity restriction, regular diet, follow up in two to three weeks with regular physician.*

✕ Notes

1. "RLL pneumonia" 是 "right lower lobe pneumonia" 的缩写, 是指 "右下肺叶肺炎"。"lobe" 在解剖学中译为 "（脑、肺等的）叶、耳垂", 如 "ear lobe" 为 "耳垂", "肝叶" 为 "lobes of liver", "脑叶" 为 "cerebral lobe"。

2. "COPD" 是 "chronic obstructive pulmonary disease" 的缩写, 是指 "慢性阻塞性肺疾病"。"pulmonary" 是指 "肺部的, 肺的", 肺动脉可表示为 "pulmonary artery"。

3. "CHF" 是 "congestive heart failure" 的缩写, 是指 "充血性心力衰竭"。"failure" 在医学英语中翻译为 "衰竭", 如肾脏衰竭表示为 "kidney failure", 肝脏衰竭表示为 "liver failure"。

4. "ABGs" 是 "arterial blood gases" 的缩写, 是指 "动脉血气"。动脉血气分析是指对溶解于动脉血液中气体成分（O_2、CO_2 等）的分压和含量进行测定, 从而了解的通气功能, 呼吸衰竭与严重程度, 以及各类型的酸碱失衡状态。

5. "ceftriaxone" 译为 "头孢曲松"。"azithromycin" 译为 "阿奇霉素"。"steroid" 译为 "类固醇"。

🎧 **Task 3 Listen to a conversation between a patient and a nurse, then fill into the blanks.**

听力6.1

Mr. John, a patient with heart surgery, will be discharged. Jessica, a ward nurse, is giving him some instructions.

1. Mr. John is feeling _____ now, and he is going to be discharged _____ .

2. Dr. Smith has written _____ for Mr. John.

3. There are _____ suggestions for Mr. John to tell what to do at home.

4. Mr. John should go to the hospital _____ and see a doctor as soon as the illness _____ .

✎ Notes

1. "surgery" 意为 "外科手术"，"heart surgery" 译为 "心脏手术"。

e. g. This lady had laser surgery on her eyes last year.

这位女士去年做了眼部激光手术。

2. "ward" 意为 "病房，病室"，"ward nurse" 译为 "病房护士"。此外还有 clinic nurse（门诊护士）、community nurse（社区护士）、obstetric nurse（助产护士）、attending nurse（随访护士）、special care nurse（特护护士）、critical care nurse（危重病护士）等。

Task 4　**Listen the conversation again. In pairs, talk about the advice that Jessica gave Mr. John. Then fill the blanks.**

听力 6.1

Eating habits	1. Have (1) _____ diet, avoid (2) _____ , greasy, indigestible food. 2. Do not eat too much each time. 3. Develop a regular and (3) _____ diet.
Living habits	1. Avoid any (4) _____ and have enough rest. 2. Give up (5) _____ and drinking. 3. Do not (6) _____ when taking a bath.
Taking medicines	1. Take (7) _____ before each meal, three times a day. 2. When feeling (8) _____ or cardiac discomfort, just put a piece of this lozenge under tongue and don't swallow it.

✎ Notes

1. And Dr. Smith has written a discharge certificate for you.

史密斯医生给你写了出院证明。

句中 "certificate" 意为 "证明，证明书"，"discharge certificate" 译为 "出院证明"，由主治医生开具，是证明病人经住院治疗已经出院的证明书，内容没有出院小结详细。

2. When you feel chest pain or cardiac discomfort, just put a piece of this lozenge under your tongue and don't swallow it.

当你感到胸痛或心脏不适时，只需在舌头下放一片这种含片，不要吞咽。

句中 "cardiac" 意为 "relating to the heart" 表示 "与心脏有关的"，可译为 "心脏的"，"cardiac discomfort" 表示 "心脏不适"。

e. g. The doctor managed to revive the injured worker with cardiac massage.

医生通过心脏按压使受伤的工人苏醒了过来。

句中 "lozenge" 表示 "锭剂，含片"。

e. g. Do you have any cough syrup or lozenges?

请问你们这儿有止咳糖浆或含片吗？

Task 5   Work in groups, make a dialogue between a nurse and a patient with the following information. Swap roles and practice again.

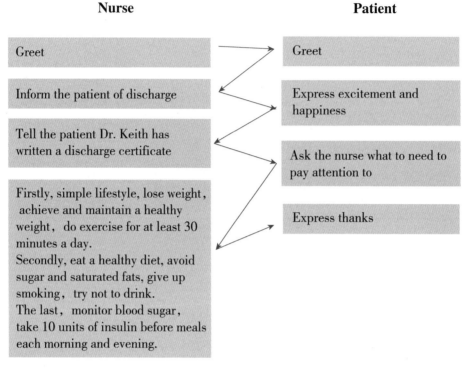

Nurse

Greet

Inform the patient of discharge

Tell the patient Dr. Keith has written a discharge certificate

Firstly, simple lifestyle, lose weight, achieve and maintain a healthy weight, do exercise for at least 30 minutes a day.
Secondly, eat a healthy diet, avoid sugar and saturated fats, give up smoking, try not to drink.
The last, monitor blood sugar, take 10 units of insulin before meals each morning and evening.

Patient

Greet

Express excitement and happiness

Ask the nurse what to need to pay attention to

Express thanks

Communication Tips：

Authentic oral expression in discharge

Some oral English is always used when providing service or help for patients in discharge. Besides the common expressions, do you know any more authentic expressions?

We often say	What else can we say
You are going to be discharged tomorrow.	1. You are allowed to be discharged from hospital tomorrow. 2. You will be discharged from hospital tomorrow.
Even if you're discharged, you still need to take a rest at home.	1. Remember to have a rest at home, though you're discharged. 2. You must also have a good rest after leaving the hospital.
I'm here to talk over the discharge with you.	1. I want to discuss something about leaving hospital. 2. I'd like to discuss the discharge from hospital.
This is the discharge order for you.	1. I have written a discharge order for you. 2. Here is the discharge order for you.
Pay attention to the post-hospital care.	1. Pay attention to the patient care after leaving the hospital. 2. Be careful of the patient care after discharge.

Listening and Speaking

Activity 2　Giving Instructions to Patients – 2
（Exercise，Recheck and Discharge Procedure）

Task 1　When making discharge plan, six aspects need to be considered. Work in pairs, match the items (1 – 6) to their specific contents (a – f).

1. Medication	a. It provides continuous care and drug monitoring for patients who need to be transferred to community care.
2. Residence	b. It provides life guidance, work and rest, diet and other suggestions for discharged patients.
3. Follow-up Community Care	c. It should be documented the instructions about dosage, times and any special instructions – such as the need to take the drugs with food or milk.
4. Activities of Daily Living	d. It teaches patients basic knowledge of disease identification and prevention and other precautions after discharge.
5. Follow-up Physical Health Care	e. It can help give patients the basic support they need to remain in the community or stay at home.
6. Education, Financial Assistance, and Other Needs	f. It makes rehabilitation training plan, work and rest time and intensity for discharged patients to ensure the patients recover as soon as possible.

Notes

Discharge planning is the process of transitioning a patient from one level of care to the next. It is a personalized description provided to patients when they move from hospital to home, or to follow-up healthcare providers when they move to a longer-term care facility.

出院计划是将患者从一个护理级别转移到下一个护理级别的过程。它是在患者从医院回到家中时提供给他们的个性化说明，或者在他们移送到长期护理机构时提供给后续医疗保健机构的说明。

Task 2　Listen to the conversation and fill in the blanks.

The nurse, Daisy, is making rounds. Mr. King wants to be discharged soon. So he is asking Daisy when he can be discharged.

听力 6.2

Mr. King：Excuse me, Daisy. What does the doctor say about me?

（1）_____?

Daisy：Dr. Miller has examined your case and current situation. He said （2）_____ and can （3）_____ in this afternoon. Congratulations!

Mr. King：That's great. Thank you. I'm so excited. （4）_____, and I've been looking forward to going home （5）_____.

Daisy：Your wish will come true soon.

✎ **Notes**

1. Dr. Miller said you were well recovered. 米勒医生说你恢复得很好。

此句中, "recover" 意为 "恢复健康, 康复, 痊愈", "you were well recovered" 表示 "你恢复得很好"。

e. g. The brave mother has fully recovered from the accident.

这位勇敢的妈妈已经从那次车祸中完全恢复过来。

2. I've been looking forward to going home for a long time. 我盼望回家很长时间了。

此句中, "looking forward to doing sth." 表示盼望做某事。

e. g. I'm looking forward to returning to my job as a ward nurse as soon as possible. 我盼望尽早回到病房护士的工作中。

🎧 **Task 3 Listen to the conversation and answer the following questions.**

听力6.3

Mr. King will be discharged this afternoon. Daisy is giving him some discharge instructions.

(1) What's on the medication list?

_____

_____

_____

(2) What kind of exercise can Mr. King do after a week?

_____

_____

_____

(3) Is Mr. King suitable for some aerobic exercises? Why?

_____

_____

_____

(4) Where is Mr. King going to take the bill? And how can he pay for it?

_____

_____

_____

(5) Does Mr. King need to go back to the hospital for checkup? If yes, what time?

_____

_____

_____

✎ **Notes**

1. There's also a medication list, containing the dosage of drugs and precautions. 还有一个药物清单, 里面有药物的剂量和注意事项。

此句中 "dosage" 通常指 " (药的) 剂量, 用量, 服药量", "the dosage of drugs" 即为 "药物的剂量"。

e. g. His attending doctor prescribed him a high dosage of vitamin C.

他的主治医生给他开了大剂量的维生素 C。

2. About a month later, you can do some aerobic exercises.

一个月后，你可以做一些有氧运动。

此句中"aerobic"意为"有氧的，有氧健身的"，"aerobic exercises"即为"有氧运动"，是指人体在氧气充足供应的情况下进行的体育锻炼，其运动时间一般为 30 分钟或以上，强度在中等或中上的程度。这种锻炼，氧气能充分燃烧体内的糖分，还可消耗体内脂肪，增强和改善心肺功能，预防骨质疏松，调节心理和精神状态，是健身的主要运动方式。

3. They can improve muscle oxygen transport capacity and improve your cardiopulmonary function. 这些运动可以提高肌肉运氧能力，改善你的心肺功能。

此句中"cardiopulmonary"是由词根"cardio"+"pulmonary"构成的合成词。"cardio"表示"心"，"pulmonary"表示"肺"，"cardiopulmonary"即为"心肺"，"cardiopulmonary function"表示"心肺功能"。

大部分医学词汇是由前缀，词根，后缀构成的。利用构词法记忆医学词汇会有事半功倍的效果。例如："peri-"（前缀：表示周围）+"card"（词根：表示心脏）+"itis"（后缀：表示炎症）="pericarditis"（心包炎）

🎧 **Task 4**　**Listen the conversation again. In pairs, talk about the discharge instructions that Daisy gave Mr. King. Match the items to the suggestions.**

听力 6.3

1. Medication	a. can't do exercise at once
	b. do light exercises
2. Exercise	c. take at the doctor's office
	d. the dosage and precautions
3. Discharge procedure	e. review in two weeks
	f. stay at home and gradually increase the walking time
4. Recheck	g. pay in cash or check
	h. telephone communications
	i. do aerobic exercises

✂ **Notes**

1. discharge instructions：出院指导，是指出院回家后，为促进安全和适当的护理连续性而向患者或监护人提供的任何形式的文件。出院指导包括饮食、用药、活动与休息、定期复查、特别指导、功能锻炼、再次就医等内容。做好出院指导，对患者出院后的康复和提高生活质量具有极其重要的意义。

2. Recheck：再次诊治，复诊。

凡是到医院接受检查、诊断和治疗的都称为病人。病人可分为住院病人与门诊病人。门诊病人中又有初诊病人和复诊病人。初诊病人，医学上定义为"伴有初诊行为的病人"；复诊病人即不伴有初诊行为的病人，也就是在初诊之后继续到医院诊治的病人。初、复诊的概念是以疾病为依据的。病人患了任何一种急性病，第一次到医院门诊就诊时，叫做初诊，此时医院就计算为一个新病例；下次续诊时，即为复诊。

Task 5 Use Task 3 as a guide. In pairs, practice giving advice to discharged patient. Use the following prompts to help you.

Advice forDischarged Patient		
sports	can't get back to exercise right away	
	do some light exercises	
	do some aerobic exercises	
bill	take at the doctor's office	
	pay in cash or check	
checkup	come back for checkup in two weeks	
	contact at 6734521	

Communication Tips:

Blessing of discharged patients

The patient is about to recover and leave hospital. What kind of blessing should we send? Here are some best wishes for discharged patient.

1. Good health, good luck, longevity, happiness.

2. Your recovery is my happiness; your health is my peace. You'll be all right.

3. Health is the greatest happiness in life. Your health concerns all the friends. I wish you a speedy recovery and laughter.

4. May health and happiness surround you like the sun shining on the earth, and may luck and happiness drift around you like the spring rain moistening all things.

5. Disease in you, pain in me, I wish you an early recovery. My happiness comes from your health. I will always bless you, happiness will always accompany you around.

Listening and Speaking

Activity 3   Making a Referral of a Patient

Task 1 Select the information needed for a patient referral form from the information below.

a. patient's name, phone number and address	g. physician's homecare orders
b. diet precautions	h. patient's social context
c. patient's discharge date and summary	i. medication records
d. patient's medical history	j. hospital transfer summary
e. patient's physical condition	k. patient's education information
f. patient's work experience	l. patient's property status

Needed information：_____

✎ Notes

Referral of a patient is a written request from one medical professional to another medical professional or medical service provider. A patient referral form mainly includes the following information：patient's personal information, diet precautions, medical history, physical status, discharge information, homecare orders, doctor's information, medication records and transfer summary, etc.

病人转诊是一名医疗专业人员向另一名医疗专业人员或医疗服务机构提出的书面请求。病人转诊表主要包括以下信息：患者的个人信息，饮食注意事项，病史，身体状态，出院信息，家庭护理医嘱，医生信息，用药记录和转院小结等。

🎧 **Task 2　Listen to the conversation and answer the following questions.**

听力 6.4

Susan, a ward nurse, is calling Martin, a district nurse, to discuss Selena's referral to the District Care Service Center.

（1）Why did Susan call Martin?

_____

_____

_____

（2）What's the matter with Selena?

_____

_____

_____

（3）What's Selena's condition now?

_____

_____

_____

（4）Who is Selena's GP?

_____

_____

_____

（5）What kind of food can Selena eat? And how much food can she eat for each meal?

_____

_____

_____

✎ Notes

1. "district nurse" 意为 "a nurse who visits patients in their homes"，即 "上门护理病人的护士"，可译为 "社区护士，片区护士"。

e. g. After John was discharged, the district nurse came to change the bandages for him each day.

约翰出院后，社区护士每天来给他换绷带。

2. Who is her GP? 她的家庭医生是谁?

此句中 "GP" 是 "general practitioner" 的缩写,意为 "全科医生",又称 "家庭医生",是执行全科医疗的卫生服务提供者,也是健康管理服务的主要提供者。全科医生一般是以门诊形式处理常见病、多发病及一般急症;社区全科医生工作的另一个特点是上门服务,全科医生常以家访的形式上门处理家庭的病人,根据病人的不同情况建立各自的家庭病床和各自的医疗档案。

3. She had a stroke about a month ago, causing hemiplegia in the right side of her body.

她一个月前中风了,导致她右侧身体偏瘫。

此句中 "stroke" 表示 "中风",又称 "脑卒中",是一种急性脑血管疾病,是由于脑部血管突然破裂或因血管阻塞导致血液不能流入大脑而引起脑组织损伤的一组疾病。"have a + 疾病" 表示 "患……病","had a stroke" 就是 "患了中风"。

e. g. My daughter has a headache, feel nauseous and keep vomiting.

我女儿头痛,觉得恶心和不停地呕吐。

"hemiplegia" 表示 "偏瘫,半身麻痹",在中医中表示 "半身不遂",是指同一侧上下肢、面肌和舌肌下部的运动障碍,是急性脑血管病的常见症状。

4. She still needs to eat some soft food that is easy to digest.

她仍然需要吃一些容易消化的软食。

此句中 "soft food" 译为 "软食",指婴儿或病弱者吃的软而烂的食物或半流质性的食物。

e. g. You can only eat soft food within a week, such as soft-boiled eggs, oatmeal, milk and toast.

一周内你只能吃软食,如煮得嫩嫩的鸡蛋、燕麦粥、牛奶和烤面包。

Task 3 According to the two nurses' conversation, decide whether the following sentences are correct or not. Put a "T" to the correct ones and an "F" to the incorrect ones.

□ (1) Selena will be referred to Tongji Hospital for some district care services.

□ (2) Selena lives in a red roofed house and her daughter usually looks after her.

□ (3) Selena had a stroke, causing hemiplegia in her left-sided body.

□ (4) Selena can't stand steadily, and needs to be prepared a walking frame.

□ (5) Selena's discharge summary will be sent to the Care Service Center tomorrow.

Notes

1. district care service:译为 "地区护理服务",是整个卫生保健系统不可或缺的组成部分,为家庭环境或卫生中心诊所内的人们提供护理和其他支持。地区护理人员与每位客户、他们的护理人员和其他医疗专业人员密切合作,提供专业和协调的护理,同时促进独立性。

2. a walking frame:(伤残人士使用的)助行架,也称 "步行器",一般用铝合金材料制成,是一种三边形(前面和左右两侧)的金属框架,自身很轻,可将患者保护在其中,有些还带脚轮。步行器可以支持体重便于站立或步行,其支承面积大。

听力 6.4

Task 4   Listen to the conversation again, and complete the patient referral form below. Work in pairs, discuss your answers.

DISTRICT CARE SERVICE CENTER

PATIENT REFERRAL FORM

Patient Information

Name: (1)_____   **Gender:** Male / (Female)   **Age:** (2)_____

Phone number: (3)_____

Address: 141 Central Street, Heping District

Guardian's name: Lucy   **Phone number:** (4)_____

Clinical Information

GP: (5)_____   **Referred by:** Susan

Place of referral: Tongji Hospital

Diagnosis Information

1. (6)_____   **2.** right-sided hemiplegia

3. inarticulate, difficulty swallowing   **4.** (7)_____

5. (8)_____   **6.** (9)_____

Care and Diet Information

Care:

1. help in life

2. help in the bath

3. help use walking frame

Diet:

1. (10)_____

2. 50 mg for each meal

Task 5 **A hemiplegia patient will be referred to the District Care Service Center. Use Task 4 as a guide, practice the patient referral communication between a ward nurse and a district nurse according to the form below.**

DISTRICT CARE SERVICE CENTER
PATIENT REFERRAL FORM

Patient Information

Name: Hyman   **Gender:** (Male)/ Female   **Age:** 56

Phone number: 18689732648

Address: 1101 Huaihai Road, Baiyun District

Guardian's name: Mike   **Phone number:** 18638463951

Clinical Information

GP: John Smith   **Referred by:** Helen

Place of referral: The First People's Hospital

Diagnosis Information

1. right-sided hemiplegia	2. speech indistinct
3. difficulty in swallowing	4. walking unstable
5. limbs are not under control	6. difficulty in defecation

Care and Diet Information

Care:	Diet:
1. help in daily life	1. balanced and digestible food
2. turn over every 2 hours	2. ban high sugar and irritating food
3. keep body clean	

👥 Communication Tips:

Referring a patient by telephone

After discharge, some patients need to be referred to the district care center for further care. At this time, ward nurses often need to refer with district nurses by telephone. Here are some common expressions.

1. District Care Service. This is ... speaking!

2. Hello, it's ... here from ...

3. Wait a minute, let me get areferral form.

4. I've got ... I need to refer to you for some district care services. Could I give you some conditions now?

5. Yes, I'm ready. It was ..., wasn't it?

6. OK. What's the patient's name?

7. Do you have...'s phone number, please?

8. Could you please repeat that?

9. What is wrong with...?

10. How do we take care of ... diet?

Writing

If you are Nurse Susan in Activity 3 Task 4, please write a patient referral letter to District Nursing Service Center in order to introduce Patient Selena's condition.

Patient Referral Letter

Date: 21/09/2020

To: District Nursing Nurse,

District Nursing Service Center, 124 High Street, Dongshan District.

Subject: referral of patient's care to District Nursing Service Center

Dear Sir/Madam,

I am writing with regards to the referral of _____ _____

_____

_____

_____

_____

_____

_____

_____

_____

_____

_____

Do contact me if you require any clarifications of the case.

Thank you.

Yours sincerely,

Susan

Proverbs and Sayings

❖ Careful care can really prevent the epidemic.

　悉心的护理才能真正避免疾病的流行。

❖ Careful nursing, enthusiastic service and patient's health are our persistent pursuit.

　用心护理，热情服务，病人的健康是我们执着的追求。

❖ A doctor or nurse should not pass in front of the wounded.

　一个医生或护士是不应该在伤员面前昂首而过的。

书网融合……

　　听力材料6.1　　　听力材料6.2　　　听力材料6.3　　　听力材料6.4

Unit 7 Facilitating Patients' Rehabilitation

PPT

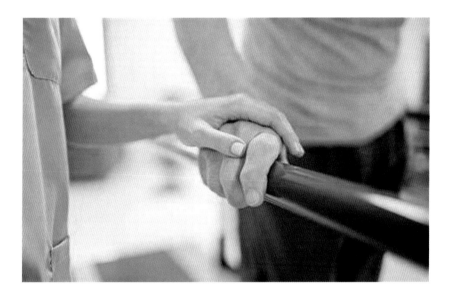

Learning Objectives

Reading part:

Be able to identify the details of different types of rehabilitation.

Listening and Speaking part:

1. Be able to identify and recognize specific information on main ADLs.

2. Be able to apply the tips to incorporate empathy in nursing, using effective communication strategies for showing empathy to patients.

3. Be able to identify and recognize specific information on the medical terms of ROM exercise.

4. Be able to give relevant explanations on ROM exercise prior to providing healthcare, using communication tips for some simple instructions.

5. Be able to assist patients in setting goals for overcoming depressing and helping them with rehabilitation.

6. Be able to apply communication tips to praise for patients' strengths and recovery progress.

Writing part:

Be able to write a patient's record according to the ROM assessment result, using appropriate medical terminology, accurate grammar and punctuation.

Warm – up Exercises

Susan is a patient who is in traction after a road accident. She needs to do exercises for her neck, ankle, and knee. Can you help her to label the different types of ROM exercises and choose the appropriate ones?

shoulder adduction	neck extension	knee bend	ankle pump	toe raise
shoulder abduction	ankle rotation	elbow flexion	wrist stretch	

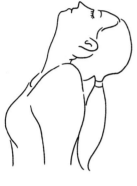

A _____

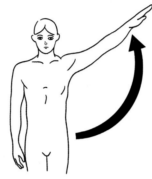

B _____

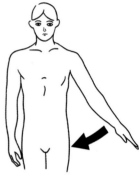

C _____

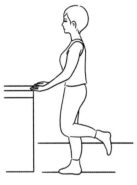

D _____

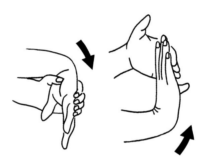

E _____

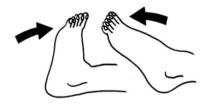

F _____

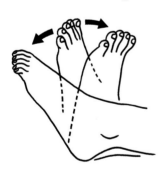

G _____

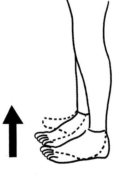

H _____

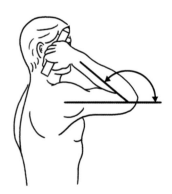

I _____

阅读译文

Reading

A Guide to Different Types of Rehabilitation

There are many types of rehabilitation therapy, each designed to address specific ranges of issues. What they all have in common is their primary goals: to help individuals recover from illness, injury, surgery, stroke, cardiac events or other medical issues and regain functional abilities and independence lost to these events. Here we'll outline several types of rehabilitation therapy commonly used in treatment plans designed to meet those goals.

Physical Therapy

This type of rehabilitation therapy works to improve movement dysfunction. Therapists work with patients to restore movement, strength, stability and/or functional ability and reduce pain via targeted exercise and a range of other treatment methods.

Occupational Therapy

This form of therapy focuses on restoring an individual's ability to perform necessary daily activities. This may mean working to improve fine motor skills, restore balance, or assist patients in learning how to increase their functional ability via use of adaptive equipment.

Speech Therapy

This type of rehabilitation therapy is used to address difficulties with speech, communication and/or swallowing.

Respiratory Therapy

Used to aid patients who have breathing disorders or difficulties, this form of rehabilitation therapy works to help them decrease respiratory distress, maintain open airways and, when necessary, learn how to use inhalers and supplemental oxygen properly.

Cognitive Rehabilitation

Also commonly called cognitive – behavior rehabilitation, this type of therapy works with patients to improve memory, thinking and reasoning skills.

Vocational Rehabilitation

This form of therapy is geared towards preparing individuals to return to work after an injury, illness, or medical event.

Each type of rehabilitation therapy can be accessed in various healthcare settings. These include inpatient rehabilitation facilities, outpatient rehabilitation clinics and home – based rehabilitation services.

Inpatient rehabilitation centers typically offer all of these common types of therapy and others, along with medical/nursing care, provided by a multidisciplinary team of rehabilitation professionals in a hospital – type setting. Outpatient clinics vary in the types of therapy they offer, and those services are offered by appointment, with patients traveling to their offices for therapy sessions. Home – based rehabilitation programs typically offer a few basic services – usually physical, occupational, and speech therapies – in a patient's home, with therapists visiting by appointment.

When multiple types of therapy are needed to aid an individual in recovery and rehabilitation or close medical supervision is necessary, seeking services in an inpatient facility is generally recommended as the safest and most efficient means of treatment. Outpatient or home – based services may be most appropriate for patients who need fewer services or less intensive medical/rehabilitative care.

(419 words)

✎ Notes

1. There are many types of rehabilitation therapy, each designed to address specific ranges of issues.

康复治疗有多种类型，每一种都旨在解决特定范围的问题。

本句"address"应翻译为"解决；处理"。

e. g. We must address ourselves to the problem of traffic pollution.

我们必须设法解决交通污染问题。

文章提到六种康复治疗类型，其中最重要的三种是：Occupational Therapy, Physical Therapy and Speech Therapy. Occupational therapists provide occupational therapy treatments to help individuals who require specialized assistance to participate in everyday activities. Physical therapists provide treatment for those who are experiencing pain or difficulty in functioning, moving or living life normally. Speech therapy can help treat a wide variety of issues involving language, communication, voice, swallowing and fluency.

职业疗法，物理疗法和言语疗法。职业治疗师提供职业治疗，以帮助需要专业帮助的个人参与日常活动。物理治疗师为那些在正常活动或生活中经历疼痛或困难的人提供治疗。言语治疗可以帮助治疗多种问题，包括语言，交流，声音，吞咽和流利度等问题。

2. This form of therapy focuses on restoring an individual's ability to perform necessary daily activities.

这种治疗形式侧重于恢复个人进行必要的日常活动的能力。

"focus on"集中于；侧重于

e. g. Something that also stimulates your brain. So you just don't focus on small things or small challenges.

有一些能激发你大脑的东西。所以你不要只关注小事情或小困难。

"necessary daily activities"是指"必要的日常活动"，such as eating, dressing, brushing one's teeth, completing school activities and working.

3. Used to aid patients who have breathing disorders or difficulties, this form of rehabilitation therapy works to help them decrease respiratory distress, maintain open airways and, when necessary, learn how to use inhalers and supplemental oxygen properly.

这种形式的康复疗法用于帮助有呼吸障碍或困难的患者，可帮助他们缓解呼吸窘迫，保持呼吸道畅通，必要时学习如何正确使用吸入器和补充氧气。

"Used to aid patients who have breathing disorders or difficulties"过去分词短语做定语，修饰"this form of rehabilitation therapy"。

"respiratory distress"是指"呼吸窘迫"，英文解释是"a medical term that refers to both difficulty in breathing, and to the psychological experience associated with such difficulty, even if there is no physiological basis for experiencing such distress."

Acute Respiratory Distress Syndrome 急性呼吸窘迫综合征

e. g. She was brought to Siloam Gleneagles Hospital, on 28 June, where she died with respiratory distress 20 days after onset.

6月28日，她被送往 Siloam Gleneagles 医院，发病20天后死于呼吸窘迫。

4. Outpatient or home – based services may be most appropriate for patients who need fewer services or less

intensive medical/rehabilitative care.

门诊康复诊所或以家庭为基础的康复服务机构可能最适合需要较少服务或非重症医疗/康复护理的患者。

"be appropriate for" 适合于

e. g. Although laparoscopic anti – reflux surgery has many benefits, it may not be appropriate for some patients.

尽管腹腔镜手术治疗胃食管反流病有很多优点，但还是有部分病人不适合做该手术。

"intensive care" （医院里的）特别护理；重症监护，英文解释是 "continuous care and attention, often using special equipment, for people in hospital who are very seriously ill or injured."

"less intensive medical/rehabilitative care" 这里指 "非重症医疗/康复护理"。

After – reading Exercises

Task 1　Match the words with their proper meaning.

1. rehabilitation	a. 心脏事件
2. stroke	b. 认知康复
3. cardiac events	c. 言语疗法
4. Physical Therapy	d. 康复
5. dysfunction	e. 呼吸疗法
6. Occupational Therapy	f. 中风
7. Speech Therapy	g. 物理疗法
8. Respiratory Therapy	h. 呼吸窘迫
9. Cognitive Rehabilitation	i. 功能紊乱
10. respiratory distress	j. 职业疗法

Task 2　Complete the following sentences with a word or short phrase from the text.

1. There are many types of rehabilitation therapy, each ＿＿＿＿＿＿＿＿ to address specific ranges of issues.

2. This form of therapy ＿＿＿＿＿＿＿ restoring an individual's ability to perform necessary daily activities.

3. This form of therapy is ＿＿＿＿＿＿＿＿ preparing individuals to return to work after an injury, illness, or medical event.

4. Outpatient clinics ＿＿＿＿＿＿＿ in the types of therapy they offer, and those services are offered by appointment, with patients traveling to their offices for therapy sessions.

5. Outpatient or home – based services may be most ＿＿＿＿＿＿＿ for patients who need fewer services or less intensive medical/rehabilitative care.

Task 3　In pairs, discuss the following questions.

1. Can you tell the differences between physical therapy and occupational therapy? what are they?

_____

_____

2. If a patient needs physical therapy, respiratory therapy and cognitive rehabilitation for his/her recovery, which type of healthcare setting is generally recommended and why?

_____

_____

Listening and Speaking

Activity 1　Assessing Activities of Daily Living（ADLs）

Task 1　Please label the pictures with the words in the box.

bedpan	commode	shower chair
walking frame	walking stick	urinal bottle

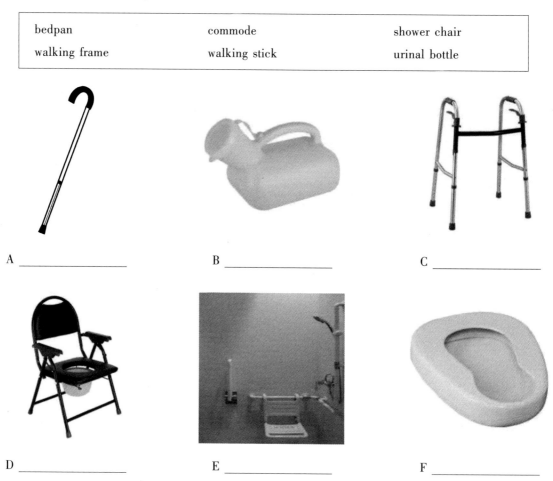

A _____　　B _____　　C _____

D _____　　E _____　　F _____

✎ Notes

Activities of daily living（ADLs or ADL）is a term used in healthcare to refer to people's daily self-care activities. Health professionals often use a person's ability or inability to perform ADLs as a measurement of their functional status, particularly in regard to people post injury, with disabilities and the elderly.

日常生活活动（ADLs 或 ADL）是医疗保健中使用的一个术语，指的是人们的日常自我保健活动。卫生专业人员经常使用一个人执行 ADL 的能力或无能力来衡量他们的功能状态，特别是对于受伤后的人、残疾人和老年人。

Task 2　**Listen and complete the ADL assessment for patients 1 ~ 3 in the table. Write** *independent* **or** *dependent* **for each ADL.**

听力 7.1

ADLs	1. **Karl**	2. **Ellen**	3. **Selina**
washing	*independent*		
dressing			
grooming			
oral hygiene			

✎ Notes

1. My hands are shaky and it's difficult to hold the razor stably without cutting myself.

我的手在颤抖，很难拿稳剃刀不伤到自己。

2. Ring the buzzer when you're ready and I'll give you a hand. 当你准备好时请按呼叫器，我会来帮你的。

"ring the buzzer" 是指按响床旁呼叫器，也可以用 "press the nurse call/button" 来表示。

3. My back hurts when I bend down, but I can't put my tights on without bending down.

我弯腰的时候背就会疼，但不弯腰就穿不上衣服。

Task 3　**The Complaint Board criticized the nurse for not showing empathy towards her patient. Read it and answer the following questions.**

I'm Karl's daughter. My father suffers from early dementia and requires assistance with simple tasks. In general, the staff is kind and helpful, but he often complains about Nurse Susan. She is often too busy to help my father and sometimes refuses to help him to eat. According to my father, Nurse Susan is very impolite, treats him like a child and complains about him to other patients. Quote "I'm not paid enough to clean up stupid, old men like Karl." I visited my father on 24 May at 9：30 am. He was crying, he had not had a shave or a wash and his breakfast tray was still on the table. He hadn't eaten anything. He seemed confused and was very uncomfortable. I find this situation totally unacceptable and I ask the center to investigate this case thoroughly.

1. What's wrong with the patient Karl?

_____

_____

2. Which ADLs does Karl need help with?

_____

_____

3. What is the daughter's complaint about?

_____

_____

4. How does Nurse Susan feel about her job?

_____

_____

5. What advice would you give to Nurse Susan?

_____

_____

Notes

dementia: a serious mental disorder caused by brain disease or injury, that affects the ability to think, remember and behave normally. 痴呆；精神错乱

Task 4 **Listen to three nurses talking to their patients. How much empathy do they demonstrate? and put a tick (√) in the column.**

听力7.2

	no empathy	a little empathy	a lot of empathy
Nurse 1			
Nurse 2			
Nurse 3			

Notes

1. Empathy is seeing, understanding, and sharing others' viewpoints without judgment. Important in nurses' relationships with patients and their quality of care, empathy improves nurses' performance in the following areas: establishing respect; encouraging positive behavior and attitudes; making ethical decisions; gathering medical history information; accurately administering medicine.

同理心是看到、理解和分享他人的观点而不加判断。同理心在建立良好的护士与病人之间的关系，提高护理质量中起着至关重要的作用，主要体现在以下几个方面：建立尊重；鼓励积极的行为态度；伦理决策；收集病史信息；精准给药。

2. Tips toincorporate empathy in nursing:

● Listen to patients and show curiosity about their lives;

● Be kind and respectful;

● Develop cultural competence and awareness;

● Use self – care strategies to prevent compassion fatigue;

● Lead by example.

在护理中融入同理心的技巧：

● 倾听病人，对他们的生活表现出好奇心；

● 友善和尊重他人；

● 培养文化能力和文化意识；

● 使用自我护理策略来防止同情疲劳；

● 以身作则。

Task 5   Use Task 4 as a guide, practice communicating with a patient who is having chemotherapy and try to supply assistance.

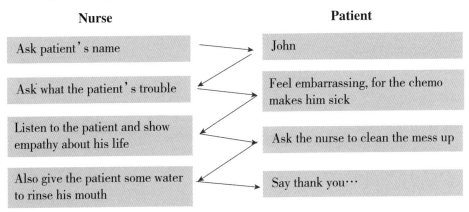

Nurse	Patient
Ask patient's name	John
Ask what the patient's trouble	Feel embarrassing, for the chemo makes him sick
Listen to the patient and show empathy about his life	Ask the nurse to clean the mess up
Also give the patient some water to rinse his mouth	Say thank you…

Communication Tips:

Patient's emotions and grief are important and need to be acknowledged and accepted: show empathy.

Empathy is the ability to imagine yourself in the position of another person and so to share and understand that person's feelings.

Showing empathy	➤ I know/understand exactly how you feel.
	➤ I can see it's difficult for you.
Reassuring	➤ Please don't worry. Let me clean you up and you'll feel much better.
	➤ It can happen to anyone. Don't be embarrassed.
	➤ I'm used to it; it's part of my job.
Respecting the patient's privacy	➤ Do you want me to come back later?
	➤ I'll bring a screen to put around the bed. You can have a little privacy.

Listening and Speaking

Activity 2   Measuring a Patient's Range of Motion (ROM)

Task 1   Look at illustrations A – E and write the medical terms in the box.

rotation	abduction	adduction	extension	flexion

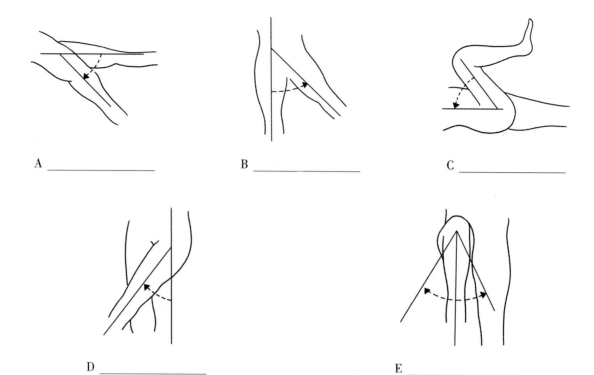

A _____   B _____   C _____

D _____   E _____

✎ Notes

1. Range of motion exercise refers to activity aimed at improving movement of a specific joint. This motion is influenced by several structures: configuration of bone surfaces within the joint, joint capsule, ligaments, tendons, and muscles acting on the joint. 关节活动度练习是指旨在改善特定关节运动的活动。这种运动受多种结构的影响：关节内骨表面的构造、关节囊、韧带、肌腱和作用于关节的肌肉。

2. extension: act of stretching or straightening out a flexed limb 伸展

3. flexion: the action of bending sth. 屈曲

4. rotation: the action of an object moving in a circle around a central fixed point 旋转

5. abduction: moving of a body part away from the central axis of the body 外展

6. adduction: moving of a body part toward the central axis of the body 内转

Task 2 **Listen to the conversation between Nurse (N) and Mr. Davis (D), a patient, and then answer the following questions.**

听力7.3

1. How does Mr. Davis feel this morning?

_____

_____

2. What does he think about the old exercises?

_____

_____

3. Does he start with the left or right leg?

_____

_____

4. What does he think of the new exercises?

_____

_____

Notes

We use **prepositions of movement** to say in which direction something is moving.

我们使用移动介词来表示某物朝哪个方向运动。

e. g. Lift **up** your arm above your head. 将手臂举过头顶。

Push **down** with your hand. 用手压下去。

Move your leg **to** the side / **to** the left / **to** the right.

将你的腿移向一侧/向左/向右。

Task 3   Read Nurse Susan's assessment of Bill Smith, who is in traction after a road accident. Match the words in bold to definitions 1 ~ 6.

FRIENDSHIP REHABILITA-TION	**ROM Assessment**: **Bill Smith**, *27yrs*
	patient conscious but tired, *with nausea*; *left shoulder*, *bruising and swelling*
	ROM **limited** to 100 with great **discomfort**
	left leg **immobilized**; other joints fully **mobile**
	health status prior to accident excellent; patient unwilling to perform ROM
	Planning ROM exercises
	Stage 1: begin with **passive ROM** two times a day (9:00, 17:00) for first two days.
	Stage 2: teach patient to perform **active ROM** three times a day (9:00, 12:00, 17:00).

1. prevented from moving _____

2. exercises the patient can do by himself / herself _____

3. able to move normally _____

4. a feeling of pain or of being physically uncomfortable _____

5. prevented from increasing beyond a particular point _____

6. exercises a nurse does for the patient _____

Notes

1. passive ROM: therapist or equipment moves the joint through the range of motion with no effort from the patient 被动性关节活动

2. active ROM: patient performs the exercise to move the joint without any assistance to the muscles surrounding the joint 主动性关节活动

Task 4 **Listen and tick "✓" the ROM exercises the patient can do in 1 ~ 6, and circle the correct words in 7 ~ 10.**

听力 7.4

Flow sheet – ROM（range of motion exercises）		
Patient：Bill Smith **Room No.**：Bed 34 **Date**：18/06/2021 **Time**：9 a. m.		
Movement	**Result**	**Comments**
R shoulder flexion	1. _____	WNL
R shoulder rotation	2. _____	WNL
R elbow extension	3. _____	7. WNL with <u>some / no</u> pain
R elbow flexion	4. _____	8. WNL with <u>some / no</u> pain
L shoulder flexion	5. _____	9. limited to <u>100° / 120°</u>
L shoulder extension	6. _____	10. <u>able / not able</u> to do
Nurse's initials	GPR	

✎ **Notes**

WNL：within normal limits 强调在能力正常范围内；而 WFL，是指"within functional limits"，强调在功能正常范围内。

Task 5 **Read the following case and play a nurse and a patient based on the flow sheet. In the dialogue, you should complete the following tasks.**

Tasks：

1. Guide the patient John Smith through ROM exercises.

2. Praise the patient for his strength and recovery progress.

Flow sheet – ROM（range of motion exercises）		
Patient：John Smith **Room No.**：Bed 39 **Date**：21/07/2021 **Time**：9：00 a. m.		
Movement	**Result**	**Comments**
R knee bend	✓	WNL
R leg extension	✓	limited to 120°
R leg abduction	✓	WNL with some pain
R ankle pump	✓	WNL
Nurse's initials	KPR	

📖 **Communication Tips**：

Health professionals should always give relevant explanations and education prior to providing healthcare.

Regular exercises are important to assist patients in recovering. The following sentences in the language box are some simple instructions which are recommended for exercises of patients' ankle, leg and knee.

	➢ In bed, slowly push your foot up and down. Repeat several times a day. ➢ You can do this exercise immediately after surgery.
	➢ Move your ankle in a circular motion. ➢ Repeat five times in each direction, three or four times a day.
	➢ Keep your heel on the bed and bend your knee. Then straighten your leg again. ➢ Repeat ten times, three or four times a day.
	➢ Stand up and life your knee, but not too high. ➢ Hold for two or three seconds. Repeat ten times, three or four times a day.
	➢ Move your leg out to the side as far as you can and then back. ➢ Repeat ten times, three or four times a day.

Listening and Speaking

Activity 3　Setting Goals and Giving Encouragement

Task 1　What are the patients in illustrations A ~ C thinking? Match sentences 1 ~ 3 to patients A ~ C.

1. I just want to take a walk by myself.

2. One of my goals is to be able to eat by myself.

3. I hope I can already put on my shoes by myself.

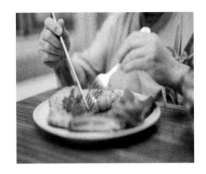
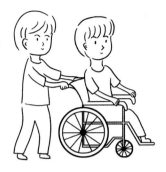
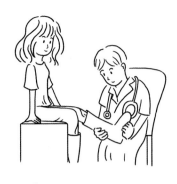

A _____   B _____   C _____

Notes

Setting goals can not only impact mental health, but it can also help the patient overcome depression and help him/her with rehabilitation. If a nurse sets goals that are only his/her idea, the patient will be less likely to comply. Allow patients to contribute to their goals.

设定目标不仅可以影响心理健康，还可以帮助患者克服抑郁，帮助康复。如果护士设定的目标只是他/她的个人想法，病人就不太可能遵守。允许患者参与自己康复目标的制定。

Task 2 **Put the words in 1 – 6 in the correct order to make sentences. Then listen to the three patients in the passage and check your answers.**

听力 7.5

1. what's / goal / long – term / your / ?

_____

2. you / want / today / to do / what / do / ?

_____

3. you / what / do / can / ?

_____

4. three sets of ten / for today / on each arm / our goal is

_____

5. that / can / you / do / ?

_____

6. this exercise / three times / do / a day / can you / ?

_____

Notes

physio: physical therapy or physiotherapy is the health care profession primarily concerned with the remediation of impairments and disabilities and the promotion of mobility, functional ability, quality of life and movement potential through examination, evaluation, diagnosis and physical intervention. It is carried out by physical therapists and physical therapist assistants.

物理治疗，是一种主要通过检查、评估、诊断和物理干预，对损伤和残疾进行修复，以改善行动能力、功能能力、生活质量和运动潜力的医疗保健行业。它由物理治疗师和物理治疗师助理进行。

Task 3   Listen to the conversation between Nurse (N) and Alisa (A). Pay attention to the nurse's expressions of encouragement and comforting words used in the conversation, and put a tick (✓) in the column.

听力 7.6

	1. It doesn't matter. / Never mind.
	2. I can really understand that you…
	3. Please come back to see the doctor for check - up in two weeks.
	4. You did a good job. / You did really well.
	5. Don't worry.
	6. Don't be nervous. Your doctor is an expert for this disease.
	7. You will recover soon.
	8. I could see that was hard work for you, but you did a good job.

❈ Notes

But your body needs the nutrition so that you can regain your strength and energy.

但是你的身体需要营养，这样你才能恢复你的体力和能量。

Task 4   Listen to a nurse working with Tracy, a patient, on her recovery exercises. Are these sentences *true* (T) or *false* (F)?

听力 7.7

1. (T / F) Tracy's goal is four sets of ten on each leg.
2. (T / F) It is more difficult to move the left leg.
3. (T / F) The nurse asks Tracy to do leg lifts.
4. (T / F) Tracy repeats the exercise three times on the left leg.
5. (T / F) Tracy says she's in a lot of pain.

❈ Notes

1. Our goal is three sets of ten on each leg.

我们的目标是每条腿练习三组，每组十次。

2. Move your leg out to the side as far as you can. 腿尽可能地朝一个方向伸。

Task 5   Use Task 4 as a guide, practice communicating with a patient who needs to do exercises for his/ her fingers and toes. Follow these steps and

➢ explain the benefits of the exercise.

➢ set the goals.

➢ encourage the patient.

Language Tips：

When + clause + it helps	
We use ***when + clause + it helps*** to explain the benefits of exercise to a patient.	***When I hold your head*** , ***it helps*** your neck.
	When you bend your fingers , ***it helps*** the muscles in your wrist.
	When you touch your toes , ***it helps*** the muscles in your back.
	When you do your exercises , ***it helps*** you recover from surgery.

Communication Tips：

Praise patients for their strengths and recovery progress.

Patients typically feel anxious about their illness process, they may lose confidence in their own strengths or the positive recovery gains. Praising could remind them of these facts.

Setting goals	Let's see what you can do today. Our goal is three sets of ten on each leg. What do you think?
	One of your goals is to be able to eat by yourself.
	What do you want to do today?
	It's important to do these exercises every day for your recovering.
Giving encouragement	It's much better than yesterday. Let's try again.
	Long stay in bed may make you lose confidence. But you are really doing such a good job of recovering.
	You're doing very well. Try it again… Good job!
	You have done very well considering the extent of your injuries. I have noticed that you have fought to recover in such a determined way.

Writing

Read Nurse Susan's assessment of Bill Smith, who is in traction after a road accident. Please write a patient's record according to the ROM assessment result.

FRIENDSHIP REHABILITATION	*ROM Assessment*：*Bill Smith*, *27yrs* patient：conscious but tired, with nausea; left shoulder, bruising and swelling ROM limited to 100 with great discomfort left leg immobilized; other joints fully mobile health status prior to accident excellent; patient unwilling to perform ROM
	Planning ROM exercises Stage 1：begin with **passive ROM** two times a day （9：00, 17：00）for first two days. Stage 2：teach patient to perform **active ROM** three times a day （9：00, 12：00, 17：00）.

Proverbs and Sayings

✧ Movement is a medicine for creating change in a person's physical, emotional, and mental states.

运动是改变一个人的身体、情感和精神状态的良药。

✧ Wherever the art of Medicine is loved, there is also a love of Humanity.

哪里有人爱医学艺术，哪里就有人爱人性。

书网融合……

 听力材料 7.1   听力材料 7.2   听力材料 7.3   听力材料 7.4

 听力材料 7.5   听力材料 7.6   听力材料 7.7

Unit 8　Community Care

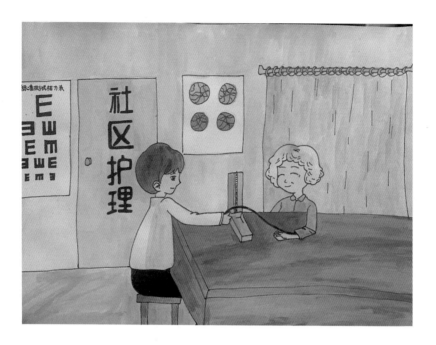

Learning Objectives

Reading part：

Learn some knowledge about community care.

Listening and Speaking part：

1. Be able to identify and recognize specific information on community nursing.

2. Be able to explain nutrition and diseases to the elderly, using effective communication strategies with patient in community.

3. Be able to explain the precautions for medications to the elderly.

4. Be able to teach patients how to take medicine safely.

5. Be able to identify and recognize specific information about community health nursing.

Writing part：

Be able to write a short essay about the community health nursing, using appropriate medical terminology, accurate grammar and punctuation.

Warm – up Exercises

Match the English expressions with the pictures on the current social hot phenomena.

Delay retirement retirement	Pension insurance	Community – based elderly care
Aging population	Empty – nest elderly	To pay filial respects for one's parents parents

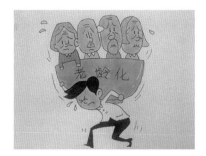

A _____

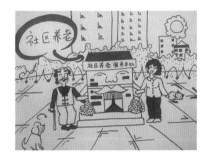

B _____

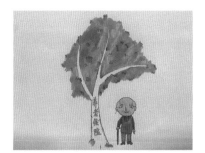

C _____

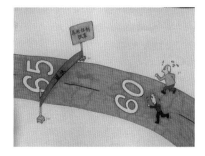

D _____

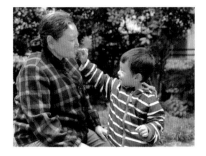

E _____

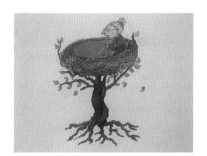

F _____

阅读译文

Reading

The Nurse's Role in Community Health

In the past, caregivers journeyed on horseback to the homes of their neighbors to provide medical services. These caregivers were crucial to reducing the mortality rates in their communities. As time went on, hospitals were built. This began the implementation of organized healthcare. Today, nurses practice in a variety of settings and community health is again re-emerging as an integral part of providing care to everyone.

What is Community Health Nursing?

A community is a group of people in aspecific location, which includes places where people live, work and go to school. Community health nursing is commonly practiced in geographic locations like cities and rural areas.

Community health nursing is a discipline that incorporates evidenced – based research along with advances in science and new approaches for improving the health. The practice takes into consideration the cultural and socioeconomic backgrounds of the people in the community to ensure appropriate interaction and sensitivity when working with them.

What is the Goal of Community Health Nursing?

The goal of community health nursing is to promote, protect and preserve the health of the public. Community health nursing involves these basic concepts:

✦ Promote healthy lifestyle

✦ Prevent disease and health problems

✦ Provide direct care

✦ Educate community about managing chronic conditions and making healthy choices

✦ Evaluate a community's delivery of patient care and wellness projects

✦ Institute health and wellness programs

✦ Conduct research to improve healthcare

What is the Role of a Community Health Nurse?

The primary role of community health nurses is to provide treatment to patients. Additionally, community health nurses offer education to community members about maintaining their health so that they can decrease the occurrence of diseases and deaths. They plan educational assemblies, hand-out fliers, conduct health screenings, dispense medications and administer immunizations.

Nurses also may distribute health-related items like condoms and pregnancy tests. Examples of some health issues that community health nurses try to control or eliminate are:

✦ Infectious and sexually transmitted diseases

✦ Obesity

✦ Poor nutrition

✦ Substance abuse

✦ Smoking

✦ Teen pregnancy

Where do Community Health Nurses Work?

Community health nurses work in hospitals, community centers, clinics, school sand government health agencies. Community health nurses are important to regions where healthcare is not easily accessible because they can travel to remote places and isolated areas of a city.

Community health nurses have the ability to improve the welfare of individuals and their communities. They are at the forefront of bringing quality patient care to the most vulnerable and underserved members of society.

(435 words)

✂ Notes

1. These caregivers were crucial to reducing the mortality rates in their communities. 这些护理人员对降低其社区的死亡率起到了至关重要的作用。

本句中 "be crucial to doing sth." 翻译为 "对 ... 至关重要"。

e. g. This medicine is crucial to treating the disease. 这种药物对治疗这个疾病至关重要。

2. Today, nurses practice in a variety of settings and community health is again re-emerging as an integral part of providing care to everyone.

今天，护士在各种环境中工作，社区卫生再次成为为每个人提供护理的一个组成部分。

本句中 "practice" 译为 " （医生或律师的）业务活动，工作"，如：

clinical practice 诊所工作

medical practice 医务工作

3. Community health nursing is a discipline that incorporates evidenced – based research along with advances in science and new approaches for improving the health. 社区健康护理是一门结合循证医学研究、先进科学和改善健康新方法的学科。

evidenced – based research 循证医学研究。循证医学研究就是医疗决策（即病人的处理，治疗指南和医疗政策的制定等）应在现有的最好的临床研究依据基础上做出，同时也重视结合个人临床经验的相关研究。

4. The practice takes into consideration the cultural and socioeconomic backgrounds of the people in the community to ensure appropriate interaction and sensitivity when working with them. 为了确保服务社区居民时能做到良好的互动和恰当的体贴，社区护理工作必须考虑到社区居民的文化和社会经济背景。

5. Educate community about managing chronic conditions and making healthy choices. 教育社区成员管理好慢性病和做出健康的选择。

"chronic conditions" 又称 "chronic disease" 是指 "慢性病"，与它对应的是急性病 "acute disease"。急性就是发病突然，进展快，变化大，甚至很快危及生命或者是死亡。如急性阑尾炎等疾病。慢性就是发病缓慢，隐匿，不容易被发现，变化慢，进展慢等特点。如慢性阑尾炎，慢性胃炎等。

6. "sexually transmitted diseases"（STD）性传播疾病或性传染疾病，又称性病，是指主要通过性接触、类似性行为或间接接触传播的一组传染病我国目前重点防治的 STD 共 8 种，即梅毒、淋病、艾滋病、软下疳、性病性淋巴肉芽肿、非淋菌性尿道炎、尖锐湿疣和生殖器疱疹，其中前 3 种属于《中华人民共和国传染病防治法》规定管理的乙类传染病，其他 5 种为卫生部规定需作监测和疫情报告的病种。

After – reading Exercises

Task 1　Match the words with their proper meaning.

1. Mortality Rate	a. 实施
2. Implementation	b. 社区健康护理
3. Discipline	c. 死亡率
4. Evidenced – based Research	d. 循证研究
5. Community Health Nursing	e. 营养不良
6. Chronic Conditions	f. 未成年人怀孕
7. Administer Immunizations	g. 学科
8. Obesity	h. 肥胖
9. Poor Nutrition	i. 接种疫苗
10. Teen Pregnancy	j. 慢性病

Task 2　Complete the following sentences with a word or short phrase from the text.

1. _____ were crucial to reducing the mortality rates in their communities.

2. _____ is commonly practiced in geographic locations like cities and rural areas.

3. Nurses also may distribute health – related items like _____ .

4. The primary role of community health nurses is to _____ .

5. Community health nurses work in hospitals, _____ , clinics, schools and _____ .

Task 3　In pairs，discuss the following questions.

1. What is the goal of community health nursing?

_____

_____

2. Why are community health nurses important to regions where healthcare is not easily accessible?

_____

_____

Listening and Speaking

Activity 1　Talking about Nutrition for the Elderly

Task 1　Match the following English words about nutrition（1～10）with the Chinese（a～j）.

Nutrients	
1. fat	a. 蛋白质
2. calory	b. 脂肪
3. protein	c. 热卡（能量）
4. dietary fiber	d. 维生素
5. vitamin	e. 碳水化合物
6. carbohydrate	f. 叶酸
7. calcium	g. 食物纤维
8. folic acid	h. 铁
9. iron	i. 矿物质
10. mineral	j. 钙

Task 2　Match the following diseases（1～8）with corresponding nutrient deficiency or excessive intake of nutrients（a～h）.

Disease	Nutrient deficiency or excessive intake of nutrients
1. osteoporosis	a. vitamin A deficiency
2. high blood pressure	b. calcium deficiency
3. fatty liver	c. iron deficiency
4. nyctalopia	d. excessive sodium intake
5. iron – deficiency anemia	e. excessive fat intake
6. beriberi	f. vitamin B_1 deficiency
7. bleeding gums	g. lack of dietary fiber
8. constipation	h. vitamin C deficiency

Notes

营养缺乏症（nutritional deficiency）是生物有机体由于摄入营养素不足如维生素缺乏、蛋白质缺乏、微量元素不足而引起各种疾病症状。

e. g. The most common nutritional deficiency is lack of dietary iron.

最常见的营养缺乏是膳食中铁的不足。

Task 3　Listen to the conversation and decide if they are true or false. Write "T" for true or "F" for false.

听力 8.1

1. Older patients are likely to develop poor eating habits for many reasons.	
2. Having difficulty getting to a supermarket or standing long enough to cook a meal for old patients is one reason for their poor eating habits.	
3. Nutrition can have little impact on well – being and independence.	
4. Liquid nutrition supplements can replace solid food.	
5. The elderly are advised to take an appropriate amount of multivitamins and minerals.	

Notes

Not only can supplements not replace a healthy and balanced diet, but nutrition from food is more beneficial to the body thanvitamins and minerals from nutritional supplements. 营养补充剂不仅不能取代健康均衡的饮食，而且食物中的营养比营养补充剂中的维生素和矿物质对身体更有益。

营养补充剂（nutrient supplements），又称营养补充品、营养剂、饮食补充剂等，是作为饮食的一种辅助手段，用来补充人体所需的氨基酸、微量元素、维生素、矿物质等。

e. g. The protein left over would be dried into a powder and used as a nutrient supplement. 将剩下的蛋白质干燥成粉末，用来做营养添加剂。

Task 4　listen to a dialogue between a nurse and a patient, then fill the blanks.

听力 8.2

Healthy life style involves keeping a ＿＿＿＿＿＿ , living a ＿＿＿＿＿＿ and undertaking ＿＿＿＿＿＿ . One must have some basic ideas about ＿＿＿＿＿＿ and find the best way for the nutrients to work out for the body.

Notes

They refer to careful calculations on proteins, vitamins and calories.

他们指的是对蛋白质、维生素和卡路里的仔细计算。

Task 5 A patient wants to consult the nurse because of bad appetite. Make a dialogue with the information given below.

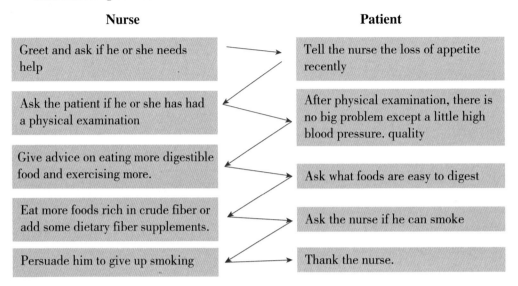

Nurse	Patient
Greet and ask if he or she needs help	Tell the nurse the loss of appetite recently
Ask the patient if he or she has had a physical examination	After physical examination, there is no big problem except a little high blood pressure. quality
Give advice on eating more digestible food and exercising more.	Ask what foods are easy to digest
Eat more foods rich in crude fiber or add some dietary fiber supplements.	Ask the nurse if he can smoke
Persuade him to give up smoking	Thank the nurse.

Communication Tips:

Some tips on how to communicate with older patients in ways that are respectful and informative.

Strategies	Examples
Use Proper Form of Address	You might ask your patient about preferred forms of address and how she orhe would like to address you. Use Mr. , Mrs. , Ms. , and so on.
Make Older Patients Comfortable	Ask staff to make sure patients have a comfortable seat in the waiting room and help with filling out forms if necessary. Be aware that older patients mayneed to be escorted to and from exam rooms, offices, and the waiting area.
Take a Few Moments to Establish Rapport	Introduce yourself clearly. Show from the start that you accept the patient and want to hear his or her concerns.
Try Not to Rush	Avoid hurrying older patients. You can say: "Take your time, don't worry."
Avoid Interrupting	By speaking more slowly, you will give them time to process what is being asked or said. If you tend to speak quickly, especially if your accent is different from what your patients are used to hearing, try to slow down.
Use Active Listening Skills	Face the patient, maintain eye contact, and when he or she is talking, use frequent, brief responses, such as "okay," "I see," and "uh – huh."

Listening and Speaking

Activity 2   Applying Home Medication Management for Seniors

Task 1   Match the medicines（1～5）with the right methods of taking the medicines（a～e）.

Medicine	Methods
1. Penicillin	a. You can buy and take it without a prescription, if you cough badly.
2. Cough syrup	b. A skin test is necessary before taking the medicine.
3. Herb medicine	c. Apply the medicine directly to the affected area.
4. Rheumatic plaster	d. Put the medicine into a pot, add some cold water, simmer gently for 20 mins, and drain the solution. Do the same step three times.
5. Vitamin C effervescent tablets	e. When people want to use them, the medicine can be dropped into water or another fluid to make a solution.

Notes

Effervescent Tablets 是指泡腾片。泡腾片在我国是一种较新的药物剂型，与普通片剂不同，泡腾片利用有机酸和碱式碳酸（氢）盐反应做泡腾崩解剂，置入水中，即刻发生泡腾反应，生成并释放大量的二氧化碳气体，状如沸腾，故名泡腾片。

泡腾片的正确服用方法，取半杯凉开水或温开水（100～150ml），将一次用量的药片投入杯子中，等气泡完全消失、药物全部溶化后，再摇匀服下。

Task 2   Listen to the conversation and answer the following questions.

听力 8.3

（1）What's wrong with the patient?

_____

_____

（2）Does the patient have a prescription?

_____

_____

（3）Can the patient buy any penicillin without a doctor's prescription?

_____

_____

（4）What medicine did the nurse recommend to the patient?

_____

_____

（5）Can the patient buy the vitamin C effervescent tablets without a doctor's prescription?

_____

_____

Notes

Are you allergic to any type of medication?

你对某种药品过敏吗？

药物过敏反应也称药物变态反应（drug allergic reaction），是由药物引起的过敏反应，是药物不良反应中的一种特殊类型，与人的特异性过敏体质相关，仅见于少数人。随着医药卫生事业的发展，本病有增多的趋势，其预防要引起医生和患者本人的高度重视。药物过敏反应一般发生于多次接触同一种药物后，首次发病具有潜伏期，再次发病则可即刻发生。它的发生由于异常的免疫反应所致。这种反应总得来说都是对人体不利的。

　　e. g. Dairy products may provoke allergic reactions in some people.

乳制品可能会引起某些人的过敏反应。

听力 8.3

Task 3　Listen to the conversation again and complete the following blanks.

The patient wanted to buy some ＿＿＿＿＿＿（1）but he can't buy it without the ＿＿＿＿＿＿（2）The nurse recommended the patient to use ＿＿＿＿＿＿（3）because it can be bought in most pharmacies. The nurse reminded the patient not to take this medicine ＿＿＿＿＿＿（4）It must be dissolved in water before taking it. ＿＿＿＿＿＿（5）consumption are bad for the health.

Notes

青霉素（Penicillin，或音译盘尼西林）又被称为青霉素 G、peillin G、盘尼西林、配尼西林、青霉素钠、苄青霉素钠、青霉素钾、苄青霉素钾。青霉素是抗菌素的一种，是指分子中含有青霉烷、能破坏细菌的细胞壁并在细菌细胞的繁殖期起杀菌作用的一类抗生素，是由青霉菌中提炼出的抗生素。青霉素属于 β－内酰胺类抗生素（β－lactams），β－内酰胺类抗生素包括青霉素、头孢菌素、碳青霉烯类、单环类、头霉素类等。青霉素是很常用的抗菌药品。但每次使用前必须做皮试，以防过敏。

Task 4　Determine whether the following drugs are prescription drugs or over－the－counter drugs. If it is prescription drug, please write "Rx"; if it is over－the－counter drug, please write "OTC" in the blanks.

Drug	Rx or OTC
1. Penicillin	
2. Vitamin C effervescent tablets	
3. Cough syrup	
4. Rheumatic plaster	
5. Quick acting Jiuxin Pill	

Notes

处方药是必须凭执业医师或执业助理医师处方才可调配、购买和使用的药品；非处方药是不需要凭医师处方即可自行判断、购买和使用的药品。处方药英语称 Prescription Drug，Ethical Drug，非处方药英语称 Nonprescription Drug，在国外又称之为"可在柜台上买到的药物"（Over The Counter），简称OTC，此已成为全球通用的俗称。

　　处方药和非处方药不是药品本质的属性，而是管理上的界定。无论是处方药，还是非处方药都是经过国家药品监督管理部门批准的，其安全性和有效性是有保障的。其中非处方药主要是用于治疗各种消费者容易自我诊断、自我治疗的常见轻微疾病。

Task 5 As a nurse, you explain the effervescent tablets to patients. Use the following prompts to make a short dialogue between the nurse and the relative of a patient. Swap roles and practice again.

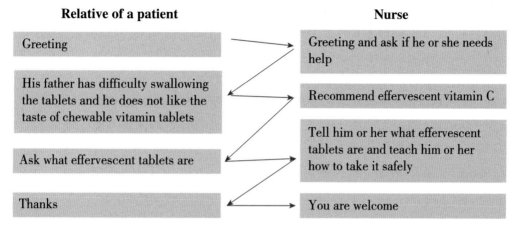

Relative of a patient	Nurse
Greeting	Greeting and ask if he or she needs help
His father has difficulty swallowing the tablets and he does not like the taste of chewable vitamin tablets	Recommend effervescent vitamin C
Ask what effervescent tablets are	Tell him or her what effervescent tablets are and teach him or her how to take it safely
Thanks	You are welcome

Communication Tips:

Use simple, clear sentences and check for understanding.

e. g: If you do not know how to use it rightly, please let me know.

Use pictures or diagrams to illustrate what you are saying.

e. g: If you still do not know how to take medicine, this picture will clearly show how to take this medicine.

Listening and Speaking

Activity 3   Introducing Community Health Service for the Elderly

Task 1 Match the English phrases (1~10) with the proper Chinese (A~J).

1	Daily care of the patient	A	压疮护理
2	Nursing diagnosis	B	对病人的日常护理
3	Bedmaking	C	护理诊断
4	Bedsore care	D	测量生命体征
5	Measurement of vital sign	E	清洗假牙
6	Denture care	F	整理床铺
7	Disinfection by ultraviolet light	G	冲洗
8	Assisting the patient to take a sit bath	H	帮助病人坐浴
9	Irrigation	I	严密隔离
10	Strict isolation	J	紫外线消毒

📝 Notes

According to the current practical experience of community nursing in China, the contents of community nursing work mainly include：①health education of community population；②To provide nursing technology and services for community families；③Prevention and control of infectious diseases and infectious diseases；④Community environment, occupational protection and home safety management；⑤Prevention and health care for children, women, middle - aged and old people in community；⑥Community population mental health and mental health care；⑦Pre hospital emergency care；⑧Hospice care and nursing.

根据目前我国开展社区护理的实践经验，社区护理工作内容主要包括：①社区人群健康教育；②为社区家庭提供护理技术与护理服务；③预防和控制传染性疾病与感染性疾病；④社区环境、职业防护与家居安全的管理；⑤社区儿童、妇女、中老年人预防保健；⑥社区人群心理卫生与精神保健；⑦院前急救护理；⑧临终关怀及护理。

🎧 Task 2   Listen to the passage and fill in the blanks.

1. Community health is the identification of _____ and the _____ and _____

of collective health within a geographically defined area.

2. Health refers to a holistic state of well - being, which includes soundness of mind, body, and _____.

3. Community health nursing is a synthesis of nursing practice and _____ applied to promoting and preserving the health of populations.

4. Health is a social, _____ and political issue.

听力 8.4

📝 Notes

1. Community health nursing is a synthesis of nursing practice and public health practice applied to promoting and preserving the health of populations.

社区健康护理是护理和公共卫生的综合，用于促进和维护人们的健康。

2. synthesis   意思是"合成，综合体"。

e. g. His work is a synthesis of several ideas. 他的作品是由几种构想综合而成的。

🎧 Task 3   Listen to the conversation and decide if they are true or false. Write "T" for true or "F" for false.

听力 8.5

☐	1. Community health nursing faces opportunities and challenges in the 21st century.
☐	2. Health refers to a holistic state of well - being.
☐	3. Community care is only for individuals.
☐	4. Health problems are closely related to society, economy and politics.
☐	5. The nursing practice and the public health practice are general and comprehensive.

📝 Notes

holistic 是指全盘的，整体的；功能整体性的。

e. g. Experts suggest a more holistic approach. 专家建议采用更全面的方法。

听力 8.5

Task 4　Listen to a conversation between Mike and Lucy and complete the blanks.

Topic	(1) **They talk about** _____.
First task	(2) The first task is to teach people how to help themselves to _____.
Conditions which may causesocial problems	(3) Alcoholism, _____, smoking, depression and _____ can lead to social problems.
The goal of community care	(4) The goal of community care is to provide a high quality service to the disabled, the elderly, the poor; attempt to improve _____; prevent _____ into care; and keep risk to a minimum.

✂ Notes

1. communicable diseases 是指传染病。

e. g. We take environmental health measures to keep off communicable diseases.

我们采取措施保护环境卫生以防止发生传染性疾病。

2. alcoholism 是指酒精中毒。酒精中毒俗称醉酒，是指患者一次饮大量酒精（乙醇）后发生的机体机能异常状态，对神经系统和肝脏伤害最严重。医学上将其分为急性中毒和慢性中毒两种，前者可在短时间内给患者带来较大伤害，甚至可以直接或间接导致死亡。后者给患者带来的是累积性伤害，如酒精依赖、精神障碍、酒精性肝硬化及诱发某些癌症（口腔癌、舌癌、食管癌、肝癌）等。

3. drug addition 是指毒瘾。毒瘾是指有嗜毒的癖好。长期应用毒品，毒品占据了受体，抑制内生性吗啡样物质合成。一旦停用，易呈现"内啡肽"缺乏，出现戒断综合征。毒品是鸦片（阿片）、海洛因、大麻和可卡因等能使人形成癖瘾的麻醉药品和精神药品，不包括烟草、酒类、安定类、安眠药及其他兴奋剂、止痛剂中的成瘾物质。

Task 5　Work in groups, use the following prompts to help you to make a dialogue between a nurse and a patient. Swap roles and practice again.

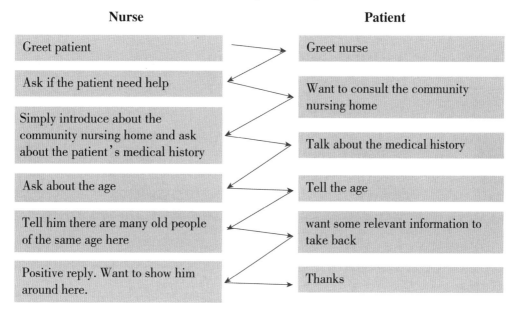

Communication Tips：

Active listening is a dynamic interactive process in which a nurse hears a clients' message, decodes its meaning and provides feedback to the client regarding the nurse's understanding of the message.

Erect posture with the upper torso slightly inclined toward the client

Direct eye contact.

Use of open, expansive gestures.

Minimal encouraging cues.

Nonverbal cues such as nodding and smiling.

Listening responses show the client that the nurse is fully present as a professional partner in helping the client understand a change in health status and the best ways to cope with it.

Body actions：smiling, nodding, leaning forward.

Writing

Write a short essay about 100 words on Community Health Nursing.

You can write the essay according to the following parts.

What is the definition of community care?

What do community health nurses mainly do?

What are thefunctions of a community health nurse?

Proverbs and Sayings

✧ Respecting patients meansrespecting oneself, and loving patients means loving hospitals.

尊重病人就是尊重自己，爱护病人就是爱护医院。

✧ Cherish life, treat others kindly and serve sincerely.

珍惜生命，善待他人，真诚服务。

✧ I wish my sincere service in exchange for your satisfactory reply, that is my greathappiness.

愿我真诚的服务换取您满意的答复，那是我莫大的幸福。

书网融合……

听力材料8.1　　听力材料8.2　　听力材料8.3　　听力材料8.4　　听力材料8.5

Unit 9   Hospice Care

PPT

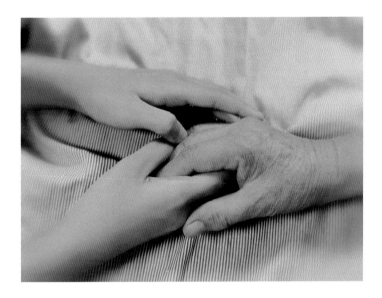

Warm – up Exercises

Hospice care is given by a team. This team is composed by the following staff. Can you match them with the correct pictures and explain what they do in hospice care?

| Physicians | Nurses | Social workers | Counselor | Clergy | Therapist |

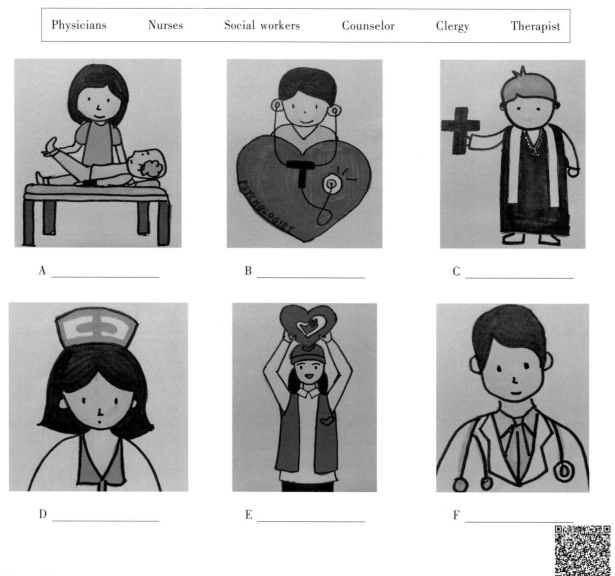

A _____

B _____

C _____

D _____

E _____

F _____

阅读译文

Reading

The Role of Hospice Nurse

Hospice care (end – of – life care) attends to the physical, emotional and sometimes spiritual needs of the terminally ill or elderly patients, focusing on palliation of their pain and symptoms, improving their quality of life and helping them die with more comfort and dignity.

Hospice care most often takes place in the patient's home or the home of a family member or friends. It also may be given in other locations, including nursing home, hospital or hospice center. Hospice care is given by a team. This team may include physicians, nurses, social workers, counselors, home health aides, clergy, therapists and trained volunteers. The team works together to give the patient and family comfort and support. A hospice nurse performs a range of duties which may include the following.

Physical care：

◇ Improving respiratory function. According to the degree of dyspnea, oxygen inhalation should be given in time.

◇ Alleviating pain——pain killer, music therapy, massage, acupuncture and moxibustion.

There are two principles for analgesic. One is Three – step Ladder Analgesic method proposed by WHO. The other is administer medication on time, not when necessary.

◇ Diet supplement. According to the patient's eating habits, give them digestible and nutritious food.

◇ Keep comfortable positions, warm and clean bodies. Help them turn over regularly to prevent bedsores.

Psychological care

◇ Through the establishment of ideas to ease the patient's fear and anxiety, so that they can feel at ease, and be full of hope and have confidence in the future of the world (after death).

Spiritual care

◇ Review of life, seeking the meaning of life, establishing the value of life. For patients who have religious faith, spiritual workers can help them find relief in religious instruction, such as immortal, paradise.

At the same time, an important aspect of the nurse's responsibility is to recognize the need to communicate with both the patient and the family, treating them as a unit of care. Hospice can also help the sick and sick family bear some fatigue and pressure.

Hospice nurses should be strong in emotion and spirit. Encountering death and serious illness on a daily basis may lead to depression and emotional fragility. Remaining stable is important not only for hospice nurses but also for patients who rely on them as sources of emotional strength during difficult times.

(384 words)

✖ Notes

1. Hospice care attends to the physical, emotional and sometimes spiritual needs of the terminally ill or elderly patients. 临终关怀是专注于满足临终患者身体、情感和精神需求的护理。

本句中"attend to"应翻译为"照料，照顾"。

e. g. The main thing is to attend to the injured. 首要任务是照顾伤者。

The staff will helpfully attend to your needs. 工作人员会帮忙满足您的需求。

2. This team may include physicians, nurses, social workers, counselors, home health aides, clergy, therapists and trained volunteers. 这支团队包括医生、护士、社工、心理顾问、家庭护工、牧师、治疗师和受过培训的志愿者。

counselor 有很多含义，"辅导员，律师，顾问"等。在本句中是"心理顾问"的意思。

e. g. The school counselor would like to see you. 学校的心理顾问要见你。

Maybe you two should go see a marriage counselor. 或许你们俩应去找个婚姻顾问做咨询。

3. Hospice can also help the sick and sick family bear some fatigue and pressure.

临终照护同时也帮助患者及其家属分担一些疲劳和压力。

"fatigue"在这里的含义是"极其疲劳"。

e. g. Reactions were slowed by fatigue. 疲劳使反应变得迟缓。

4. Encountering death and serious illness on a daily basis may lead to depression and emotional fragility. 每天面对死亡和重疾可能会产生抑郁和情绪上的脆弱。

"on a daily basis" 意思是 "每天"。

e. g. Skis are available for hire on a daily basis. 雪橇可以按天租用。

The number will change on a daily basis. 这个数字每天都会改变。

After – reading Exercises

Task 1 Match the words with their proper meaning.

1. Hospice care	a. 缓解
2. Palliation	b. 吸氧
3. Oxygen inhalation	c. 临终关怀
4. Respiratory function	d. 呼吸功能
5. Massage	e. 信仰
6. Acupuncture and moxibustion	f. 按摩
7. Bedsore	g. 针灸
8. Faith	h. 压疮
9. Dyspnea	i. 镇痛剂
10. Analgesic	j. 呼吸困难

Task 2 Complete the following sentences with a word or short phrase from the text.

1. Hospice care helps patients die with more _____ .

2. Hospice care most often takes place in the _____ home.

3. The other is administer medication _____ , not when necessary.

4. Hospice can also help the sick and sick family bear some _____ and pressure.

5. _____ is important not only for hospice nurses but also for patients who rely on them as sources of emotional strength during difficult times.

Task 3 In pairs, discuss the following questions.

1. What is hospice care?

_____

_____

_____

2. What does hospice care most often take place?

_____

_____

_____

3. How many principles are there for analgesic? What are they?

_____

_____

_____

Listening and Speaking

Activity 1　Giving Bad News

Task 1　In pairs, match the six steps of the SPIKES protocol on the right with their acronym on the left.

SPIKES—A Six – Step Protocol for Giving Bad News	
1. S—Setting up the Interview	a. 评估病人的认知
2. P—Assessing the patient's *perception*	b. 获得病人的许可
3. I —Obtaining the patient's *invitation*	c. 医学专业信息告知
4. K—Giving *knowledge* and information to the patient	d. 共情反应，稳定病人情绪
5. E—Addressing the patient's *emotions* with empathic responses	e. 策略与总结
6. S—Strategy and summary	f. 设定沟通场景

✎ Notes

The SPIKES protocol suggests six steps for delivering bad news and can be a helpful guide when nurses prepare the patient for and participate in a family meeting. It has reached guideline status in America and in a number of other countries. SPIKES is an acronym for setting, perception, invitation, knowledge, emotions and strategy and summary.

Step	Key Points
Setting	Arrange for a private room or area. Maintain eye contact. Include family or friends as patient desires.
Perception	Use open – ended questions to determine the patient's understanding. Correct misinformation and misunderstandings. Identify wishful thinking, unrealistic expectations.
Invitation	Determine how much information and detail a patient desire. Ask for permission to give results
Knowledge	Briefly summarize events leading up to this point. Use nonmedical terms and avoid jargon. Stop often to confirm understanding.
Emotions	Stop and address emotions as they arise. Use empathic statements to recognize the patient's emotion.
Strategy and Summary	Review what has been said. Set a plan for follow – up (referrals, further tests, treatment options). Offer a means of contact if additional questions arise.

在 SPIKES 模式中，将告知患者及其家属坏消息分为 6 个步骤，每一步的首字母组合成为 SPIKES。它在美国和其他一些国家已经起到了指导性作用。

步骤	要点
Setting	安排一个私密空间 保持目光交流 根据病人的意愿，允许家人或朋友在场
Perception	使用开放式问题来确定患者的对病情的了解程度 纠正误解 识别不切实际的想法
Invitation	确定患者想要了解多少信息和细节 询问是否可以告知结果
Knowledge	简要概述病情 避免使用医学术语 适当停下来确认患者对告知的理解
Emotions	使用共情话语识别患者的情绪 当患者情绪激动时，停下来安抚情绪
Strategy and Summary	回顾陈述内容 制定后续计划（转诊、进一步检查、治疗方案） 提供联系方式，以防出现其他问题

Here are some example phrases of the SPIKES protocol.

Step	Example phrases
Setting	Before we review the results, is there anyone else you would like to be here? Would it be okay if I sat on the edge of your bed?
Perception	When you felt the lump in your breast, what was your first thought? What is your understanding of your test results thus far?
Invitation	Would it be okay if I give you those test results now? Are you someone who likes to know all of the details, or would you prefer that I focus on the most important result?
Knowledge	Before I get to the results, I'd like to summarize so that we are all on the same page. Unfortunately, the test results are worse than we initially hoped. I know this is a lot of information. What questions do you have so far?
Emotions	I can see this is not the news you were expecting. Yes, I can understand why you felt that way. Could you tell me more about what concerns you?

Step	Example phrases
Strategy and summary	I know this is all very frightening news, and I'm sure you will think of many more questions. When you do, write them down and we can review them when we meet again. Even though we cannot cure your cancer, we can provide medications to control your pain and lessen your discomfort.

Task 2　In pairs, discuss the NURSE Mnemonic for Expressing Empathy and point out which technique the example phrases belong to.

N—Naming　　　　　U—Understanding　　　　R—Respecting

S—Supporting　　　　E—Exploring

Technique	Example phrases
1. (　)	①It sounds like you are worried about⋯ ②I wonder if you are feeling angry.
2. (　)	①If I understand what you are saying, you are worried you're your treatments will affect your work. ②This has been extremely difficult for you.
3. (　)	①This must be a tremendous amount to deal with. ②I am impressed with how well you have handled the treatments.
4. (　)	①I will be with you during the treatments. ②Please let me know what I can do to help you.
5. (　)	①Tell me more about your concern about the treatment side effects. ②You mentioned you are afraid about how your children will take the news. Can you tell me more about this?

Notes

the NURSE Mnemonic for Expressing Empathy

The NURSE mnemonic outlines several effective strategies for expressing empathy in difficult communication.

Naming (N) the emotion assures the patient of the nurse's recognition of his/her emotion. When the nurse uses words that communicate *understanding* (U), the patient's emotion is normalized. Communicating *respect* (R) acknowledges the patient's ability to overcome some of the challenges of his/her life – limiting illness. When a nurse uses words to communicate *support* (S), they communicate their presence at that time and in the future, assuring the patient of non – abandonment. Finally, the nurse can communicate empathy through words that *explore* (E) his/her experience. Demonstrating an interest in their narrative and the story of their experience allows patients to know the nurse is interested and to personalize their experience. In short:

- Name – name the identified emotion
- Understand – verbalize understanding of what has been said
- Respect – express respect for what the patient or family has done
- Support – assure the patient or family they will not be abandoned
- Explore – ask them to elaborate about what they are saying

表达共情的 NURSE 记忆法

表达共情的 NURSE 记忆法概述了在沟通中表达同情心的几种有效策略。首先要正确识别患者的情绪。当护士使用理解性的话语时，病人的情绪就会稳定下来。护士应表达尊敬之意，赞扬患者克服这一疾病造成不适的毅力。护士还要表达出对患者一贯的支持，以确保病人没有遗弃感。也可以通过询问患者的经历来表达同理心，对患者的叙述和经历表现出兴趣，能使患者的体验个性化。

Task 3 Listen to the conversation and complete the sentences.

听力 9.1

Harris is a 75 year old man who has just been diagnosed with advanced pancreatic cancer. Jill Campbell is his nurse in charge. Now they are discussing the illness.

1. _____ you've been feeling so tired and have no appetite.

2. At this stage _____ is not an option and _____ is important.

3. We can also start you on _____ to help with your symptoms.

4. _____ does affect the outcome.

5. _____ during the treatments.

Notes

1. advanced pancreatic cancer 晚期胰腺癌

advanced 在这里的意思是"晚期的"意思等同于 terminal。

e. g. Having a strong will to live, some patients in the terminal stage of cancer recover miraculously. 抱有强烈的生存意志，有些癌症晚期的病人奇迹般地康复了。

She worked and ran a treatment center for patients with terminal cancer. 她开了一家晚期癌症的治疗中心。

2. chemotherapy 化学疗法，化疗。"chemo –" 是指前缀，表示"化学的"；"therapy"是词根，表示"治疗"，合起来表示化学治疗，简称化疗。类似的词语还有"radiotherapy"；"radio –"是指前缀，表示"放射的"，和后面的词根合成词语放射疗法，简称放疗。

3. Your will to live does affect the outcome. 你的生存意愿会影响结果。

"the will to live" 是指生存意愿，也可用"the will to survive"代替。

will n. 意志，意图，心愿

e. g. I don't want to go against your will. 我不想违背你的意愿。

Task 4 Listen and Complete. In pairs, listen to a dialogue between a nurse and a patient, then complete the sentences and point out which technique of the NURSE Mnemonic for expressing empathy they belong to.

听力 9.2

1. (   ) You seem really _____ today.

2. (   ) I'm so _____ that you have been able to continue working while attending all of your _____ .

3. (　　) What you are doing is so ＿＿＿＿＿＿ and you are ＿＿＿＿＿＿ .

4. (　　) I know that you have been ＿＿＿＿＿＿ the pain. I will continue to work with you to ＿＿＿＿＿＿ this problem. We work together ＿＿＿＿＿＿ .

Notes

1. Unfortunately, the tumor has grown somewhat. 不幸的是，肿瘤已经有点生长了。

"tumor" 指 "肿瘤"，一般是良性的。恶性肿瘤通常用 "cancer" 来表示，也可用 a malignant (harmful) tumor 来表示恶性肿瘤。

"somewhat" 意思是 "有点，稍微"。

The situation has changed somewhat since we last met.

自我们上次见面以来情况发生了一些变化。

2. I'm so impressed that you have been able to continue working while attending all of your appointments. 你能够一边工作一边治疗，这让我深感敬佩！

"I'm so impressed that. . . " 意思是 "我深受触动，我倍感钦佩"。

e. g. I was very impressed with the talent of Michael Ball. He will go far.

我对迈克尔·鲍尔的才华印象非常深刻，他将来会前途无量。

Task 5　In pairs, make a dialogue. Use Task 1 - 2 as a guide. Use the following prompts to help you. Swap roles and practice again.

Step	Nurse	Patient
S	Ask the patient if there is anyone elsc he would like to company him before reviewing the results.	Answer the nurse's question.
P	Ask the patient's thought when he felt the lump in breast to determine the patient's understanding.	Realizethat his cancer may come back and express his nervousness.
I	Ask for permission to give results.	Agree with the nurse.
K	Summarize the condition of the patient and tell the bad news.	Response to the nurse and express his shock.
E	Express respect for what the patient has done.	Ask for the treatments.
S	Tell the treatment options and offer a means of contact.	Express his thanks.

Communication Tips：

There are several patterns of giving bad news. The common themes of them include establishing rapport in an appropriate setting, determining the patient's previous knowledge and desire for details, avoiding medical jargon, supporting patient emotions, allowing for questions, using appropriate body language, summarizing, and determining next steps.

Listening and Speaking

Activity 2　Discussing Treatments

Task 1　In pairs, discuss The WHO analgesic ladder which was released by the World Health Organization (WHO) in 1986. Then point out which step the pain belongs to.

A—Severe and persistent pain

B—Moderate pain

C—Mild pain

The Three – step Ladder		
1st step	(1)	non – opioid analgesics such as nonsteroidal anti – inflammatory drugs (NSAIDs) or acetaminophen with or without adjuvants
2nd step	(2)	weak opioids (hydrocodone, codeine, tramadol) with or without non – opioid analgesics, and with or without adjuvants
3rd step	(3)	potent opioids (morphine, methadone, fentanyl, oxycodone, buprenorphine, tapentadol, hydromorphone, oxymorphone) with or without non – opioid analgesics, and with or without adjuvants

✖ Notes

The WHO analgesic ladder was a strategy proposed by the World Health Organization (WHO), in 1986, to provide adequate pain relief for cancer patients. The analgesic ladder was part of a vast health program termed the WHO Cancer Pain and Palliative Care Program aimed at improving strategies for cancer pain management. The original ladder mainly consisted of three steps: First step, mild pain: non – opioid analgesics. Second step, moderate pain: weak opioids. Third step, severe and persistent pain: potent opioids.

1986 世界卫生组织（WTO）推荐了三阶梯止痛法，大大缓解了癌症患者的疼痛。三阶梯止痛法是世卫组织改善癌症疼痛和姑息治疗计划的一部分，旨在控制大多数癌症患者的疼痛。主要包括三个步骤：第一步，轻度疼痛：非阿片类镇痛药；第二步，中度疼痛：弱阿片类药物。第三步，严重和持续性疼痛：强效阿片类药物。

🎧 Task 2　Listen to the conversation and complete the following extracts.

In the hospice center, a nurse is talking with the patient about his treament.

We are going to continue to work at making you (1) ＿＿＿＿＿ comfortable (2) ＿＿＿＿＿.

听力 9.3

I am just (3) ＿＿＿＿＿ realizing what all of this means.

I (4) ＿＿＿＿＿ the tests and the treatments and clinic visits.

I want to (5) ＿＿＿＿＿ and let the natural course of events (6) ＿＿＿＿＿.

If these are your goals, we want to (7) ＿＿＿＿＿ that we help you to reach them.

✖ Notes

1. as + 形容词 \ 副词 + as possible "尽可能的…", 意思等同于 "as + 形容词 \ 副词 + as one can"

e. g. Please give the children as much as possible love.

请给这些孩子尽可能多的爱。

Take as much exercise as you can. 尽量多做运动。

2. have a hard time doing sth. "很难做某事"。

e. g. Having been ill in bed for nearly a month, he had a hard time passing the exam. 他在床上病了将近一个月，很难通过考试。

Task 3 Listen again. Match the sentences (1 ~ 6) with the correct communication skills (a ~ f).

听力 9.3

Sentences	**Communication Skills**
1. We will try to manage your situation and consult a dietician.	a. Respond unrealistic hopes
2. We will continue to hope for the best while also preparing for the worst.	b. Empathic statement
3. What does it mean to you?	c. Define the patient's goals of care
4. I do hope the treatment is helping you fight your cancer.	d. Exploratory question
5. If these are your goals, we want to ensure that we help you reach them.	e. State the plan of care
6. If you would like help, either I or social workers or chaplain can help you with that.	f. Provide culturally sensitive care

Notes

1. We will continue to hope for the best while also preparing for the worst.

我们要抱最大的希望，最坏的打算。

2. I want to make peace with God and let the natural course of events take place.

我想和上帝言归于好，让一切顺其自然吧。

患者说这句话的意思是接受事实，不再接受过度治疗。

3. If you would like help, either I or social workers or chaplain can help you with that. 如果你需要任何的帮助，我、社工或者牧师都能帮到你。

"chaplain"意思是"牧师"，与"pastor"（新教中对牧师的称呼，可做头衔，后面跟姓氏）意思相近；"clergy"（统称）神职人员；"priest"神父，祭司；"minister"牧师（不能用来作称呼，只描述身份）

Task 4 Listen to the conversation and answer the following questions.

A nurse is talking with a patient's son about the condition of the patient.

（1）What are the patient's symptoms?

听力 9.4

（2）What had the patient hoped?

_____

_____

（3）Does the patient's son want to give up the treatment? Why?

_____

_____

（4）What sort of care would the patient want if he was terminally ill?

_____

_____

（5）What would the patient want at the end of life?

_____

_____

_____

✖ Notes

1. My father has a high fever and slipped into a coma several times. 我父亲一直发高烧，并且昏迷了好几次了。

"slip into a coma" 意思是 "陷入昏迷"。

2. Did he discuss what sort of care he would want or would not want if he was terminally ill, e. g. tube feedings, attempted resuscitation or ventilator support?

他是否跟你们讨论过生命垂危时，他想要或不想要什么样的护理吗？比如说管饲法，尝试复苏或使用呼吸机？

Task 5 Use Task 2 & 3 as a guide, practice communicating with a patient who has a malignant tumor.

A nurse is talking with a patient about his treament.

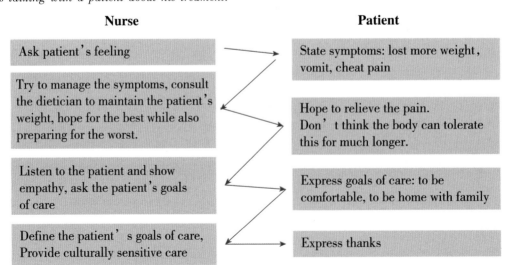

Example phrases
Could you explain what you mean?
Could you tell me what you're worried about?
Yes, your understanding of the reason for the tests is very good.
Many other patients have had a similar experience.
What do you hope for most in the next few months?
What is important to you right now?
Did he/she ever discuss what would be important to him/her at end of life from a quality – of – life point of view?

Communication Tips:

Six goals of care expressed by patients at end of life are the following:

(1) be cured

(2) live longer

(3) improve or maintain function/quality of life/independence

(4) be comfortable

(5) achieve life goals

(6) provide support for family/caregiver.

Identifying a patient's goals and helping them reach those goals may include their need to modify the goal as life draws to an end. This is a vital nursing role. The ability to sit with the patient and hear his/her grief as goals are modified and hope redefined is integral to communication in nursing care at the end of life.

Listening and Speaking

Activity 3 Supporting the Family of a Dying Patient

Task 1 Work in pairs, match the five stages of grief on the left (1 ~ 5) with their explanations on the right (a ~ e).

Five stages of grief	
1. Denial	a. Tend to deny the loss has taken place, and may withdraw from usual social contacts. This stage may last a few moments, or longer.
2. Anger	b. Try to get away from the truth in many different ways or may make bargains with God by asking, 'If I do this, will you take away the loss?'
3. Bargaining	c. When someone can no longer deny what is happening, feelings of anger, irritation, jealously and resentment arise. They put the blame on other people, colleagues, employees and counsellors. Sometimes the anger is directed at the bearer of the bad news.
4. Depression	d. Become aware of the fact that there is no more hope, they can accept the bad news.
5. Acceptance	e. Feeling numb, although anger and sadness may remain underneath. Feeling lack of control. Perhaps feeling suicidal.

✂ Notes

Elisabeth Kubler – Ross is the originator of the well – known five stages of grief. These are denial, anger, bargaining, depression, acceptance.

Stage 1   People are shocked when they receive bad news, then they will start searching for facts, the truth of for someone to blame.

Stage 2   When someone can no longer deny what is happening, feelings of anger, irritation, jealously and resentment arise. They put the blame on other people, colleagues, employees and counsellors. Sometimes the anger is directed at the bearer of the bad news.

Stage 3   At this stage, people are trying to get away from the dreadful truth in many different ways. By setting themselves goals, the blow of bad news is softened.

Stage 4   During the fourth stage, the truth is finally sinking and the person involved feels helpless and misunderstood. As a result, they will be withdrawn and avoid communications.

Stage 5   When the person involved becomes aware of the fact that there is no more hope, they can accept the bad news.

Elisabeth Kubler – Ross 是著名的"悲伤五阶段"的创始者。这五个阶段包括:拒绝、愤怒、挣扎、沮丧、接受。

第一阶段   当听到坏消息时,他们感到震惊,然后他们会开始寻找事情的真相。

第二阶段   不再否认事实,开始感到愤怒、嫉妒和怨恨。他们把责任归咎于其他人、同事、员工或顾问。有时也会指向传达坏消息的人。

第三阶段   人们正试图以不同的方式摆脱这个可怕的真相。通过为自己制定目标,坏消息的打击就被弱化了。

第四阶段   真相变得不那么重要,患者感到无助和误解。他们变得孤僻,拒绝沟通。他们不接电话或回复电子邮件。

第五阶段   当患者意识到没有希望时,他们就接受了坏消息。

听力 9.5

🎧 Task 2   Listen to the conversation and answer the following questions.

Schuberth, 56, is suffering from amyotrophic lateral sclerosis, she is losing her own ability to swallow and she has only a few days left. Her hospice nurse Jill Campbell soothes her with medicine, words, and touches.

Meanwhile, Schuberth's husband, Ken, strokes his wife's hair.

(1) What did Ken and his friends do at the party?

_____

_____

(2) What sports was Schuberth passionate about?

_____

_____

(3) What kind of person do you think Schuberth is?

_____

_____

Notes

1. amyotrophic lateral sclerosis 肌萎缩侧索硬化（ALS）也叫运动神经元病（MND）它是上运动神经元和下运动神经元损伤之后，导致包括球部（所谓球部，就是指的是延髓支配的这部分肌肉）、四肢、躯干、胸部腹部的肌肉逐渐无力和萎缩

2. occupational therapist 职业治疗师（利用特定的技能训练帮助病患者或受伤者恢复健康）

3. She was so passionate about running, cycling, and yoga. 她很喜欢跑步、骑自行车和做瑜伽。

"be passionate about" 意思是"热衷于，充满热情"。

e. g. You've got to love what you are doing and you've got to be passionate about it. 你必须爱你所做的事情，你必须对你所做的事有热情。

Task 3 Put the following statements in the correct order. Listen again and check your answers.

听力 9.5

	☐	Ken hold a party for his wife.
	☐	Schuberth specialized in swallowing disorders in children.
	☐	Schuberth told Ken she was tired and didn't want to consider using a feeding tube.
	☐	The social workers come.
	☐	Schuberth lost her own ability to eat.
	☐	Jill Campbell advise Kento take a break.

Notes

1. Her hospice nurse Jill Campbell soothes her with medicine, words, and touches. 她的临终关怀护士吉尔·坎贝尔给她用药、陪她聊天并抚摸她来减轻她的痛苦。

"soothe" 意思是"减轻，缓解，缓和（身体某部位的紧张或疼痛）"。

e. g. The music soothed her for a while. 音乐让她稍微安静了一会儿。

Muscular aches and pains can be soothed by a relaxing massage.

做放松按摩可以减轻肌肉疼痛。

Cucumber is good for soothing tired eyes. 黄瓜有助于舒缓眼部疲劳。

2. She specialized in swallowing disorders in children. 她是儿童吞咽障碍方面的专家。

"specialize" 意思是"专门研究（或从事）；专攻"。

e. g. He specialized in treatment of cancer patients. 他是治疗癌症病人的专家。

The shop specializes in hand - made chocolates.

这家商店专营手工制作的巧克力。

3. You need to make an effort to take a break every day. 你需要每天都尽力去休息一会。

"make the effort to" 意思是"尽力；尝试"。

e. g. I wish you'd make the effort to get on with her. 我希望你能试着去和她相处。

Task 4 Listen to a conversation between a nurse, Mick Harvey, and the patient's son, Ben. Then complete the following extracts.

听力 9.6

Dallas Lawson is a sixty - year - old aboriginal man who has end - stage cardiac failure and has been documented as do not resuscitate（DNR）. His whole family is present with him because they have anticipated his immi-

nent death. Michelle Harvey is the nurse caring for him and is approached by Mr. Lawson's son, Ben, in the ward corridor.

1. Dallas has _____ now. . . I'm really sorry for your loss.

2. Dad has got some brothers who _____, it might be _____ before they arrive.

3. Can you _____ him anywhere for a while?

4. You can really take _____ you need for your family to say goodbye to him.

5. I think it would _____ Mum to see him.

6. Are there any special _____ that you want us to observe while we look after his body?

7. He had such a great _____ .

🗡 Notes

1. aboriginal 澳大利亚土著的；（欧洲人到来之前某地区的人、动物等）土著的，土生土长的

2. liaison 联系；联络员；联系人

e. g. Our role is to ensure liaison between schools and parents.

我们的作用是确保学校与家长间的联系。

We work in close liaison with the police. 我们与警方密切配合。

3. sense of humor 幽默感

e. g. I can't stand people with no sense of humor. 我无法忍受毫无幽默感的人。

Task 5 Make conversations in pairs. Use Task 3 as a guide, practice communicating with a family member of a dying patient.

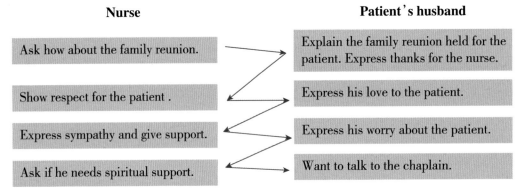

Nurse

| Ask how about the family reunion. |
| Show respect for the patient . |
| Express sympathy and give support. |
| Ask if he needs spiritual support. |

Patient's husband

| Explain the family reunion held for the patient. Express thanks for the nurse. |
| Express his love to the patient. |
| Express his worry about the patient. |
| Want to talk to the chaplain. |

📖 Communication Tips：

When treatment focus shifts from cure to comfort and quality of remaining life, the skills of listening, putting people at their ease, treating them with dignity, and providing opportunities for open and honest conversations play significant roles.

Writing

You are describing five stages of grief by Kubler – Ross Model in your language.

Proverbs and Sayings

❖ To cure sometimes, to relieve often, to comfort always.

　有时去治愈，常常去帮助，总是去安慰。

❖ Let life be beautiful like summer flowers and death like autumn leaves.

　让生如夏花之灿烂，死如秋叶之静美。

❖ Better wear out shoes than sheets.

　宁愿把鞋子穿漏，不愿把床单磨破。

书网融合……

  听力材料 9.1　　　 听力材料 9.2　　　听力材料 9.3

 听力材料 9.4　　　 听力材料 9.5　　　 听力材料 9.6

Glossary

Unit 1   Admitting Patients

accompany	/əˈkʌmpəni/	v.	be associated with 陪伴；伴随
admission	/ədˈmɪʃn/	n.	allowing or being allowed to enter or join sth 入会费；许可
attendant	/əˈtendənt/	n.	servant or companion 出席者；侍从
biopsychosocial	/baɪɒpsaɪkəˈsəʃl/	adj.	生物心理社会学的
complete	/kəmˈpliːt/	v.	finished 完成
outpatient	/ˈaʊtpeɪʃnt/	n.	a patient who does not reside in the hospital where he is being treated 门诊病人
hospitalization	/ˌhɒspɪtəlaɪˈzeɪʃ(ə)n/	n.	a period of time when you are confined to a hospital 住院治疗期
financial	/faɪˈnænʃl/	adj.	connected with money and finance 金融的，经济的，财政的，
personal	/ˈpɜːsənl/	adj.	your own; not belonging to or connected with anyone else 个人的；私人的；
physician	/fɪˈzɪʃn/	n.	a licensed medical practitioner 医生，内科医生
procedure	/prəˈsiːdʒə(r)/	n.	a way of doing sth, especially the usual or correct way （正常）程序，手续，步骤
outpatient	/ˈaʊtpeɪʃnt/	n.	a patient who does not reside in the hospital where he is being treated 门诊病人
relative	/ˈrelətɪv/	n.	a person who is in the same family as sb else 亲戚；亲属
restriction	/rɪˈstrɪkʃn/	n.	a rule or law that limits what you can do or what can happen 限制规定
resuscitation	/rɪˌsʌsɪˈteɪʃn/	n.	the act of reviving a person and returning them to consciousness 复活；
secure	/sɪˈkjʊə(r)/	v.	to protect sth so that it is safe and difficult to attack or damage 保护；保卫；使安全
shift	/ʃɪft/	v.	to move, or move sth, from one position or place to another 转移；挪动；变换；变动
stool	/stuːl/	n.	a seat with legs but with nothing to support your back or arms 凳子
stretcher	/ˈstretʃə(r)/	n.	a long piece of strong cloth with a pole on each side, used for carrying sb who is sick or injured and who cannot walk 担架

spiritual	/ˈspɪrɪtʃuəl/	adj.	connected with the human spirit, rather than the body or physical things 精神的；心灵的；宗教的
ward	/wɔːd/	n.	block forming a division of a hospital (or a suiteof rooms) shared by patients who need a similar kind of care 病房；病室

Proper names

BP	血压
HR	心率
RR	呼吸率
I. D.	身份证
OPD	门诊部

Unit 2   Administering Medications

abdomen	/ˈæbdəmən/	n.	the region of the body of a vertebrate between the thorax and the pelvis 腹部；下腹 the cavity containing the major viscera; in mammals it is separated from the thorax by the diaphragm 腹腔
administer	/ədˈmɪnɪstə(r)/	vt.	give or apply (medications) 给予（药物）
allergy	/ˈælədʒi/	n.	a medical condition that causes you to react badly or feel ill/sick when you eat or touch a particular substance 变态反应；过敏反应
amoxicillin	/əˈmɒksɪˌsɪlɪn/	n.	an antibiotic; a semisynthetic oral penicillin (trade names Amoxil andLarotid and Polymox and Trimox and Augmentin) used to treat bacterial infections 阿莫西林；羟氨苄青霉
antidote	/ˈæntidəʊt/	n.	a substance that controls the effects of a poison or disease ［药］解毒剂；解药；矫正方法
barcode	/ˈbɑːkəʊd/	n.	条形码；条码技术
capsules	/ˈkæpsl/	n.	a pill in the form of a small rounded gelatinous container with medicine inside 胶囊
contraindication	/ˌkɒntrəˌɪndɪˈkeɪʃn/	n.	a possible reason for not giving sb. a particular drug or medicaltreatment ［医］禁忌证；禁忌征候
diabetes	/ˌdaɪəˈbiːtiːz/	n.	any of several metabolic disorders marked by excessive urination and persistent thirst 糖尿病；多尿症
discomfort	/dɪsˈkʌmfət/	n.	an uncomfortable feeling of mental painfulness or distress 不适

dispense	/dɪ'spens/	vt.	give or apply (medications) (尤指在药店、药房或按处方) 配 (药); 配 (方); 发 (药)
dosage	/'dəʊsɪdʒ/	n.	the quantity of an active agent (substance or radiation) taken in or absorbed at any one time 剂量, 用量
drop	/drɒp/	n.	a small indefinite quantity (especially of a liquid) 滴
emergency	/ɪ'mɜːdʒənsi/	n.	a sudden serious and dangerous event or situation which needs immediate action to deal with it 突发事件; 紧急情况
frequency	/'friːkwənsi/	n.	the rate at whichsth. happens or is repeated 频率
high – risk	/ˌhaɪ 'rɪsk/	adj.	not safe or secure 有高风险的; 高危的
Hypoglycemia	/ˌhaɪpoʊglaɪ'siːmiə/	n.	abnormally low blood sugar usually resulting from excessive insulin or a poor diet 低血糖症; 血糖过低
infection	/ɪn'fekʃn/	n.	the invasion of the body by pathogenic microorganisms and their multiplication which can lead to tissue damage and disease 感染; 传染; 传染病
inhalation	/ˌɪnhə'leɪʃn/	n.	the act of inhaling; the drawing in of air (or other gases) as in breathing 吸入 a medication to be taken by inhaling it 吸入药剂, 雾化吸入
inhaler	/ɪn'heɪlə(r)/	n.	a dispenser that produces a chemical vapor to be inhaled in order to relieve nasal congestion 吸入器, 氧气呼吸器
injection	/ɪn'dʒekʃn/	n.	the act of putting a liquid into the body by means of a syringe 注射 any solution that is injected (as into the skin) 注射剂
insulin	/'ɪnsjəlɪn/	n.	hormone secreted by the isles of Langerhans in the pancreas; regulates storage of glycogen in the liver and accelerates oxidation of sugar in cells [生化] [药] 胰岛素
intradermal	/ˌɪntrə'dɜːm(ə)l/	adj.	situated, occurring or done within or between the layers of the skin 皮肤内的, 用于皮 (肤) 内的
intravenous	/ˌɪntrə'viːnəs/	adj.	within or by means of a vein 静脉内的
medicine	/'medɪsn/	n.	something that treats or prevents or alleviates the symptoms of disease 药; 医学; 内科
metric	/'metrɪk/	adj.	based on the meter as a standard of measurement 米制的; 公制的
nausea	/'nɔːziə/	n.	the state that precedes vomiting 恶心
omission	/ə'mɪʃn/	n.	the act of not including sb. /sth. or not doing sth. 省略, 疏忽 a thing that has not been included or done 遗漏

opioid	/əʊˈpiːɔɪd/	n.	N any of a group of substances that resemble morphine in their physiological or pharmacological effects, esp in their pain – relieving properties 阿片肽阿片类药物
patch	/pætʃ/	n.	a piece of soft material that covers and protects an injured part of the body 贴剂
pharmacist	/ˈfɑːməsɪst/	n.	a person whose job is to prepare medicines and sell or give them to the public in a shop/store or in a hospital 药剂师
pharmacy	/ˈfɑːməsi/	n.	the art and science of preparing and dispensing drugs and medicines 药房；制药业
practitioner	/prækˈtɪʃənə(r)/	n.	a person who works in aprofession, especially medicine or law（尤指医学或法律界的）从业人员
prescription	/prɪˈskrɪpʃn/	n.	an official piece of paper on which a doctor writes the type of medicine you should have, and which enables you to get it from a chemist's shop/drugstore 处方；药方
rectal	/ˈrektəl/	adj.	involving the rectum 直肠的
respiratory	/ˈrespərətri/	adj.	connected with breathing 呼吸的
sedation	/sɪˈdeɪʃn/	n.	a state of reduced excitement or anxiety that is induced by the administrative of a sedative agent 镇静，镇静作用，镇静状态
subcutaneous	/ˌsʌbkjuˈteɪnɪəs/	adj.	under the skin 皮下的
substitution	/ˌsʌbstɪˈtjuːʃn/	n.	the act, process, or substituting one thing for another 取代
suppository	/səˈpɒzətri/	n.	a small plug of medication designed for insertion into the rectum or vagina where it melts 栓剂
tablet	/ˈtæblət/	n.	a small round solid piece of medicine that you swallow 药片；片剂
tissue	/ˈtɪʃuː; ˈtɪsjuː/	n.	part of an organism consisting of an aggregate of cells having a similar structure and function 组织
topical	/ˈtɒpɪkl/	adj.	pertaining to the surface of a body part 局部的，外用的
verify	/ˈverɪfaɪ/	vt.	confirm the truth ofsth. 核实，查证

Proper names

blood sugar	血糖
carbon dioxide	二氧化碳
contact lens	隐形眼镜
Drug Enforcement Administration（DEA）	美国毒品管制局（DEA）
ID band	身份识别证

oxygen saturation	氧饱和度
PDA scanner	PDA 扫描仪
rescue agent	抢救药
reversal agent	逆转剂
side effect	副作用

Unit 3　Preventing Cross Infection

aseptic	/ˌeɪˈseptɪk/	adj.	free of or using methods to keep free of pathological microorganisms 无菌的；防感染的
bacteria	/bækˈtɪərɪə/	n.	very small living things related to plants, some of which cause disease 细菌
contaminate	/kənˈtæmɪneɪt/	vt.	to make a substance or place dirty or no longer pure by adding a substance that is dangerous or carries disease 污染；弄脏
disinfection	/ˌdisinˈfekʃən/	n.	treatment to destroy harmful microorganisms 消毒
disposable	/dɪˈspəʊzəbl/	adj.	designed to be disposed of after use 一次性的
element	/ˈelɪmənt/	n.	a simple chemical, for example oxygen or gold ［C］（化学）元素 a quality which can be noticed ［C］成分，要素
epidemic	/ˌepɪˈdemɪk/	n.	a large number of the same infectious diseases during a single period of time ［C］流行病
fundamental	/ˌfʌndəˈmentl/	adj.	forming the basis for; very important or necessary 基本的；重要的，必要的
fungi	/ˈfʌndʒaɪ/	n.	the taxonomic kingdom including yeast, molds, smuts, mushrooms, and toadstools 真菌
germ	/dʒɜːm/	n.	very small living thing which is harmful ［C］微生物；病菌，细菌
goggles	/ˈɡɒɡlz/	n.	tight – fitting spectacles worn to protect the eyes 护目镜
hygiene	/ˈhaɪdʒiːn/	n.	the science of personal and public health ［U］卫生，卫生学
inaugurate	/ɪˈnɔːɡjəreɪt/	vt.	mark the beginning of (an organization or undertaking) or open (a building, an exhibition, etc.) 为…举行仪式，为…举行落成〔开幕〕仪式
incubation	/ˌɪŋkjuˈbeɪʃn/	n.	(pathology) the phase in the development of an infection between the time a pathogen enters the body and the time the first symptoms appear 潜伏期

infection	/ɪnˈfekʃn/	n.	the act or progress of causing or getting a disease [U] 传染，感染 disease caused by a micro – organism [C] 传染病
inflamed	/ɪnˈfleɪmd/	adj.	(of a part of the body) red, sore and hot because of infection or injury 发炎的，红肿的
insert	/ˈɪnsɜːt/	vt.	to put sth into sth else or between two things 插入；嵌入
interlace	/ˌɪntəˈleɪs/	vt.	spin, wind, or twist together（使）交织；（使）组合；（使）交错
mercury	/ˈmɜːkjəri/	n.	a chemical element 汞，水银
microorganism	/ˌmaɪkrəʊˈɔːɡənɪzm/	n.	any organism of microscopic size 微生物
palm	/pɑːm/	n.	the inner surface of the hand between the base of the fingers and the wrist [C] 手掌；掌状物
pathogen	/ˈpæθədʒən/	n.	any disease – producing agent（especially a virus or bacterium or other microorganism）病原体
pneumonia	/njuːˈməʊniə/	n.	serious illness with inflammation of the lungs [U] 肺炎
rinse	/rɪns/	vt.	to remove the soap from sth with clean water after washing it 冲掉…的皂液；漂洗；清洗
rub	/rʌb/	vt.	move one thing backwards and forwards on the surface of（another）擦；搓；揉
secretion	/sɪˈkriːʃn/	n.	a liquid substance produced by parts of the body or plants [C, usually pl.] 分泌物
simultaneously	/sɪməlˈteɪniəsli/	adv.	at the same instant 同时地
sterile	/ˈsteraɪl/	adj.	free of or using methods to keep free of pathological microorganisms 无菌的
stretch	/stretʃ/	vt.	to put out an arm or a leg in order to reach sth 伸出，伸长（胳膊、腿）
susceptible	/səˈseptəbl/	adj.	likely to suffer from; defenceless 过敏的；易受…感染的
sustain	/səˈsteɪn/	vt.	keep from falling or sinking; keep up; maintain 支撑；维持；支持
swab	/swɒb/	n.	a piece of soft material used by a doctor, nurse, etc. for cleaning wounds or taking a sample from sb's body for testing（医用的）拭子，药签
tilt	/tɪlt/	vt.	to move, or make sth move, into a position with one side or end higher than the other 倾侧，使倾向于
transmission	/trænsˈmɪʃn/	n.	action or process of transmitting or being transmitted [U] 传送，传播，传达 radio or TV broadcast [C] 播送

| ultraviolet | /ˌʌltrəˈvaɪələt/ | adj. | (of light) beyond the purple end of the spectrum and unable to be seen by human beings（光）紫外的 |
| vaccination | /ˌvæksɪˈneɪʃn/ | n. | taking a vaccine as a precaution against contracting a disease 接种疫苗 |

Proper names

cross infection	交叉感染
confirmed case	确诊病例
incubation period	潜伏期
infection control	感染控制
isolation gown	隔离衣
personal protection	个人防护
suspected case	疑似病例
throat swab	咽拭子
novel coronavirus	新型冠状病毒
nucleic acid test	核酸检测

Unit 4　Preparing Patients for Radiology

angiogram	/ˈændʒioʊgræm/	n.	an X-ray representation of blood vessels made after the injection of a radiopaque substance 血管造影
ultrasound	/ˈʌltrəsaʊnd/	n.	sound that is higher than humans can hear 超声；超音 a medical process that produces an image of what is inside your body 超声波扫描检查
mammogram	/ˈmæməgræm/	n.	an examination of a breast using X-rays to check for cancer.（用于筛查乳腺癌的）乳房 X 光造影检查
diagnose	/ˌdaɪəgˈnoʊs/	v.	determine or distinguish the nature of a problem or an illness through a diagnostic analysis. 诊断（疾病）；判断（问题的原因）
interior	/ɪnˈtɪriər/	n.	the inside part of sth. 内部；里面
hyperthyroidism	/ˌhaɪpərˈθaɪrɔɪdɪzəm/	n.	a condition in which the thyroid is too active, making the heart and other body systems function too quickly.（医）甲状腺功能亢进
nausea	/ˈnɔːziə/	n.	the feeling that you have when you want to vomit, for example because you are ill/sick or are disgusted by sth. 恶心；作呕；反胃
examination	/ɪgˌzæmɪˈneɪʃn/	n.	the act of looking at or considering sth very carefully 审查；调查；考查；考察

diagnosis	/ˌdaɪəgˈnoʊsɪs/	n.	the act of discovering or identifying the exact cause of an illness or a problem 诊断；（问题原因的）判断
treatment	/ˈtriːtmənt/	n.	something that is done to cure an illness or injury, or to make sb look and feel good 治疗；诊治
diabetes	/ˌdaɪəˈbiːtiːz/	n.	any of several metabolic disorders marked by excessive urination and persistent thirst 糖尿病；多尿症
discomfort	/dɪsˈkʌmfət/	n.	an uncomfortable feeling of mental painfulness or distress 不适
radiation	/ˌreɪdiˈeɪʃn/	n.	powerful and very dangerous rays that are sent out from radioactive substances 辐射；放射线
allergy	/ˈælərdʒi/	n.	变态反应；过敏反应
injection	/ɪnˈdʒekʃn/	n.	the act of putting a liquid into the body by means of a syringe 注射 any solution that is injected (as into the skin) 注射剂
intravenous	/ˌɪntrəˈviːnəs/	adj.	within or by means of a vein 静脉内的
complication	/ˌkɑːmplɪˈkeɪʃn/	n.	a new problem or illness that makes treatment of a previous one more complicated or difficult 并发症
metformin	/ˈmetrɪk/	n.	二甲双胍；甲福明
gown	/ɡown/	n.	a piece of clothing that is worn over other clothes to protect them, especially in a hospital （尤指在医院穿的）罩衣，外罩
porter	/ˈpɔːrtər/	n.	N any of a group of substances that resemble a person whose job is to move patients from one place to another in a hospital （医院里护送病人的）护工
respiratory	/ˈrespərətri/	adj.	connected with breathing 呼吸的
breastfeeding	/ˈbrestfiːdɪŋ/	v.	When a woman breast-feeds her baby, she feeds it with milk from her breasts, rather than from a bottle. 母乳喂养
iodine	/aɪədaɪn/	n.	a chemical element. Iodine is a substance found in sea water. A liquid containing iodine is sometimes used as an antiseptic (= a substance used on wounds to prevent infection). 碘
meglumine diatrizoate			泛影葡胺；复方泛影葡胺；泛影葡胺注射剂
urticaria	/ˌɜːrtɪˈkeriə/	n.	red spots on the skin that itch (= make you want to scratch), caused by an allergic reaction, for example to certain foods. 荨麻疹
disinfect	/ˌdɪsɪnˈfekt/	vt.	to clean sth using a substance that kills bacteria. 给……消毒

diameter	/daɪˈæmɪtər/	n.	a straight line going from one side of a circle or any other round object to the other side, passing through the centre. 直径，对径
Proper names			
side effects			（药物的）副作用
contrast agent			造影剂
informed consent			知情同意
check out			核实；核查
ward nurse			病房护士
take off			脱下
in good hands			受到很好的照料（或关注）；在可靠（或内行）的人手里
breath holding			憋气；屏气

Unit 5　Caring for Operative Patients

arthroplasty	/ˌɑːθrəʊˈplæsti/	n.	surgical reconstruction or replacement of a malformed or degenerated joint［外科］关节成形术；［外科］关节造形术
aspiration	/ˌæspəˈreɪʃn/	n.	a manner of articulation involving an audible release of breath 吸入，吸入性，抽吸
analgesic	/ˌænəlˈdʒiːzɪk/	adj.	n. a medicine used to relieve pain 镇痛药 adj. capable of relieving pain 止痛的
anesthesia	/ˌænəsˈθiːʒə/	n.	loss of bodily sensation with or without loss of consciousness 麻醉
anesthesiologist	/ˌænəsˌθiːziˈɑːlədʒɪst/	n.	a specialist who administers an anesthetic to a patient before he is treated 麻醉科医师麻醉师麻醉医生麻醉学家
antibiotics	/ˌæntɪbaɪˈɑtɪks/	n.	a chemical substance derivable from a mold or bacterium that kills microorganisms and cures infections 抗生素
antihypertensive	/ˌænti, haɪpərˈtensɪv; /	adj.	a drug that reduces high blood pressure 抗高血压的
catheter	/ˈkæθətər/	n.	a thin flexible tube inserted into the body to permit introduction or withdrawal of fluids or to keep the passageway open［医］导管；导尿管；尿液管
ceftriaxone	/seftraˈɪæksn/	n.	a parenteral cephalosporin (trade name Rocephin) used for severe infection of the lungs or throat or ears or urinary tract 头孢曲松钠

drainage	/ˈdreinidʒ/	n.	emptying something accomplished by allowing liquid to run out of it 引流
extubation	/ˌekstjuːˈbeiʃən/	n.	拔管；除管法；拔除气管插管
gastric	/ˈgæstrik/	adj.	relating to or involving the stomach 胃的，胃部的
gastrointestinal	/ˌgæstrouinˈtestinl/	adj.	of or relating to the stomach and intestines 胃肠的
hypnotic	/hipˈnɑːtik/	n. / adj.	n. a drug that induces sleep 安眠药 adj. of or relating to hypnosis 催眠的
inhale	/inˈheil/	v.	draw deep into the lungs in by breathing 呼入，吸入
indwell	/inˈdwel/	v.	to exist as an inner activating spirit, force, or principle （导管、针）体内置留的
infection	/inˈfekʃn/	n.	the invasion of the body by pathogenic microorganisms and their multiplication which can lead to tissue damage and disease 感染
infusion	/inˈfjuːʒn/	n.	the passive introduction of a substance (a fluid or drug or electrolyte) into a vein or between tissues (as by gravitational force) 输液
intact	/inˈtækt/	adj.	lacking nothing essential especially not damaged fought to keep the union intact 未受损伤的
intravenous	/ˌintrəˈviːnəs/	adj.	within or by means of a vein 静脉内的
intubation	/ˌintjuːˈbeiʃən/	n.	the insertion of a cannula or tube into a hollow body organ ［临床］插管；插管法
motionless	/ˈmouʃnləs/	adj.	not in physical motion 静止的；不运动的
oozing	/ˈuːzɪŋ/	v.	渗出（ooze 的 ing 形式）；渗透
orthopedics	/ˌɔːrθəˈpiːdiks/	n.	the branch of medical science concerned with disorders or deformities of the spine and joints 骨科
osteoarthritis	/ˌɑːstiouɑːrˈθraitis/	n.	chronic breakdown of cartilage in the joints; the most common form of arthritis occurring usually after middle age 骨关节炎；骨性关节炎；关节炎
preoperative	/priˈɑːpərətiv/	adj.	happening or done before and in preparation for a surgical operation 外科手术前的；操作前的
reflux	/ˈriː, flʌks/	n.	逆流
respiratory	/ˈrespərətɔːri/	adj.	pertaining to respiration 呼吸的
sacrococcygeal	［sækrəˈkɒksidʒil］	adj.	骶尾的
saline	/ˈseiliːn/	n. / adj.	n. an isotonic solution of sodium chloride and distilled water 盐水 adj. containing salt 含盐的；咸的；含氯化钠的

scapula	/ˈskæpjələ/	n.	either of two flat triangular bones one on each side of the shoulder in human beings 肩胛；肩胛骨 复数 scapulae 或 scapulas
sedative	/ˈsedətɪv/	n. / adj.	n. a drug that reduces excitability and calms a person ［药］镇静剂 adj. tending to soothe or tranquilize 使镇静的；使安静的
solution	/səˈluːʃn/	n.	a homogeneous mixture of two or more substances 溶液
spontaneously	/spɑːnˈteɪniəsli/	adv.	without advance preparation 不由自主地
sputum	/ˈspjuːtəm/	n.	saliva mixed with discharges from the respiratory passages 痰；唾液
suffocation	/ˌsʌfəˈkeɪʃn/	n.	the condition of being deprived of oxygen（as by having breathing stopped）窒息
supine	/ˈsuːpaɪn/	adj.	lying face upward 仰卧的；掌心向上的
tracheal	/ˈtreɪkiəl/	adj.	relating to or resembling or functioning like a trachea 气管的；导管的
tract	/trækt/	n.	a system of body parts that together serve some particular purpose 道；系统；（神经纤维的）一束
urine	/ˈjʊrɪn/	n.	liquid excretory product 尿液
ventilator	/ˈventɪleɪtər/	n.	a device that facilitates breathing in cases of respiratory failure【医】呼吸机
vital	/ˈvaɪtl/	adj.	absolutely necessary 重要的；攸关生死的；非常必要的

Proper names

analgesic pump	镇痛泵
anesthesia recovery room	麻醉恢复室
blood – borne	血源性
blood vessels	血管
total knee arthroplasty	双膝关节置换术
ECG monitor	心电监护仪
general anesthesia	全身麻醉
hospitalization number	住院号码
imaging film	成像胶片
lung infections	肺部感染
medical record	病历

Patient's uniform	病号服
preoperative health education	术前健康教育
pre – operative visit	术前访视
primary nurse	责任护士
proper fixation	正确固定
respiratory rate	呼吸频率
smoking ban	禁烟
smooth drainage	输液顺畅
tracheal intubation	气管插管
urinary tube	尿管
ventilator tidal volume	呼吸机潮气量
venous access	静脉通路
vital signs	生命体征

Unit 6　Discharging Patients

aerobic	/eəˈrəʊbɪk/	adj.	based on or using the principles of aerobics 有氧的；增强心肺功能的
azithromycin	/eɪzɪθrəˈmaɪsɪn/	n.	a systemic antibacterial medicine (trade name Zithromax) that is prescribed to treat bacterial infections in many different parts of the body 阿奇霉素
cardiac	/ˈkɑːdiæk/	adj.	of or relating to the heart 心脏的；心脏病的
ceftriaxone	/seftraˈɪæksn/	n.	a parenteral cephalosporin (trade name Rocephin) used for severe infection of the lungs or throat or ears or urinary tract 头孢曲松
clinician	/klɪˈnɪʃn/	n.	a practitioner (of medicine or psychology) who does clinical work instead of laboratory experiments 临床医师
community	/kəˈmjuːnəti/	n.	a group of interdependent organisms inhabiting the same region and interacting with each other（同住一地的人所构成的）社区
dehydration	/ˌdiːhaɪˈdreɪʃən/	n.	depletion of bodily fluids 脱水
diabetic	/ˌdaɪəˈbetɪk/	n.	someone who has diabetes 糖尿病患者
district	/ˈdɪstrɪkt/	n.	a region marked off for administrative or other purposes 地区；行政区

dosage	/'dəʊsɪdʒ/	n.	a measured portion of medicine taken at any one time（通常指药的）剂量
exacerbation	/ɛksˌæsə(ː)'beɪʃən/	n.	action that makes a problem or a disease（or its symptoms）worse 加重；恶化
follow – up	/'fɒləʊ ʌp/	n.	a subsequent examination of a patient for the purpose of monitoring earlier treatment 随访
greasy	/'griːsi/	adj.	containing an unusual amount of grease or oil 多油的；油腻的
heal	/hiːl/	v.	provide a cure for, make healthy again 治愈；（使）康复
hemiplegia	/ˌhemɪ'pliːdʒɪə/	n.	paralysis of one side of the body 偏瘫；半身麻痹；半身不遂
hospitalization	/ˌhɒspɪtəlaɪ'zeɪʃ(ə)n/	n.	a period of time when you are confined to a hospital 住院治疗期
indigestible	/ˌɪndɪ'dʒestəbl/	adj.	digested with difficulty 不易消化的
infiltrate	/'ɪnfɪltreɪt/	v.	pass into or through by filtering or permeating 渗入；渗透
inhale	/ɪn'heɪl/	v.	draw deep into the lungs in by breathing 吸入（空气等）；往肺里吸
insulin	/'ɪnsjəlɪn/	n.	hormone secreted by the isles of Langerhans in the pancreas 胰岛素
lobe	/ləʊb/	n.	a somewhat rounded subdivision of a bodily organ or part（脑、肺等的）叶
lozenge	/'lɒzɪndʒ/	n.	a dose of medicine in the form of a small pellet 锭剂；含片
monitor	/'mɒnɪtə(r)/	v.	check, track, or observe by means of a receiver 监控；监视
outpatient	/'aʊtpeɪʃnt/	n.	a patient who does not reside in the hospital where he is being treated 门诊病人
physician	/fɪ'zɪʃn/	n.	a licensed medical practitioner 医生；内科医生
pneumonia	/njuː'məʊnɪə/	n.	a serious disease which affects your lungs and makes it difficult for you to breathe 肺炎
potential	/pə'tenʃl/	adj.	existing in possibility 潜在的；可能的
precaution	/prɪ'kɔːʃn/	n.	a precautionary measure warding off impending danger or damage or injury etc. 预防措施
prevention	/prɪ'venʃn/	n.	the act of preventing 预防；防止

referral	/rɪˈfɜːrəl/	n.	the act of referring（as forwarding an applicant for employment or referring a matter to an appropriate agency）转交；转送；转诊
rehabilitation	/ˌriːəˌbɪlɪˈteɪʃn/	n.	the treatment of physical disabilities by massage and electrotherapy and exercises 恢复；康复
saturated	/ˈsætʃəreɪt/	v.	infuse or fill completely 使饱和
secondary	/ˈsekəndri/	adj.	depending on or incidental to what is original or primary（疾病、感染）继发性的；第二期的
steroid	/ˈsterɔɪd/	n.	any hormone affecting the development and growth of sex organs 类固醇
stroke	/strəʊk/	n.	a sudden loss of consciousness resulting when the rupture or occlusion of a blood vessel leads to oxygen lack in the brain 中风；脑卒中
surgical	/ˈsɜːdʒɪkl/	adj.	of or relating to or involving or used in surgery 外科手术的
therapy	/ˈθerəpi/	n.	the act of caring for someone（as by medication or remedial training etc.）治疗；疗法
ward	/wɔːd/	n.	block forming a division of a hospital（or a suite of rooms）shared by patients who need a similar kind of care 病房；病室

Proper names

ABGs	动脉血气
CHF	充血性心力衰竭
COPD	慢性阻塞性肺疾病
GP	全科医生；家庭医生
iv	静脉注射
PO	口服
PT	体育；体格锻炼
RLL	右下肺叶

Unit 7　Facilitating Patients' Rehabilitation

abduction	/æbˈdʌkʃn/	n.	moving of a body part away from the central axis of the body 外展
adaptive	/əˈdæptɪv/	adj.	concerned with changing; able to change when necessary in order to deal with different situations 适应的；有适应能力的

address	/əˈdres/	vt.	to think about a problem or a situation and decide how you are going to deal with it 设法解决；处理；对付
adduction	/əˈdʌkʃən/	n.	moving of a body part toward the central axis of the body 内转
airway	/ˈeəweɪ/	n.	the passage from the nose and throat to the lungs, through which you breathe 气道
appropriate	/əˈprəʊpriət/	adj.	suitable, acceptable or correct for the particular circumstances 合适的；恰当的
commode	/kəˈməʊd/	n.	a piece of furniture that looks like a chair but has a toilet under the seat 座椅式便桶
dementia	/dɪˈmenʃə/	n.	a serious mental disorder caused by brain disease or injury, that affects the ability to think, remember and behave normally 痴呆；精神错乱
dysfunction	/dɪsˈfʌŋkʃn/	n.	(medicine) any disturbance in the function of an organ or body part 功能紊乱；机能障碍
empathy	/ˈempəθi/	n.	the ability to understand another person's feelings, experience, etc. 同感；共鸣；同情
extension	/ɪkˈstenʃn/	n.	act of stretching or straightening out a flexed limb 伸展
flexion	/ˈflekʃn/	n.	the action of bending sth. 屈曲
fracture	/ˈfræktʃə(r)/	n.	a break in a bone or other hard material（指状态）骨折，断裂，折断，破裂
grooming	/ˈɡruːmɪŋ/	n.	the things that you do to keep your clothes and hair clean and neat, or to keep an animal's fur or hair clean 打扮；装束；刷洗
inhaler	/ɪnˈheɪlə(r)/	n.	a small device containing medicine that you breathe in through your mouth, used by people who have problems with breathing 吸入器（吸药用）
inpatient	/ˈɪnpeɪʃnt/	n.	a person who stays in a hospital while receiving treatment 住院病人
intensive	/ɪnˈtensɪv/	adj.	characterized by a high degree or intensity 重症的
multidisciplinary	/ˌmʌltidɪsəˈplɪnəri/	adj.	involving several different subjects of study（涉及）多门学科的
outpatient	/ˈaʊtpeɪʃnt/	n.	a person who goes to a hospital for treatment but does not stay there 门诊病人
primary	/ˈpraɪməri/	adj.	main; most important; basic 主要的；最重要的；基本的
rehabilitation	/ˌriːəbɪlɪˈteɪʃn/	n.	the treatment of physical disabilities by massage and electrotherapy and exercises 康复

rotation	/rəʊˈteɪʃn/	n.	the action of an object moving in a circle around a central fixed point 旋转
specific	/spəˈsɪfɪk/	adj.	connected with one particular thing only 特定的
surgery	/ˈsɜːdʒəri/	n.	medical treatment of injuries or diseases that involves cutting open a person's body and often removing or replacing some parts; the branch of medicine connected with this treatment 外科手术；外科学
stability	/stəˈbɪləti/	n.	the quality or state of being steady and not changing or being disturbed in any way 稳定（性）；稳固（性）
supervision	/ˌsuːpəˈvɪʒn/	n.	management by overseeing the performance or operation of a person or group 监督，管理
swallow	/ˈswɒləʊ/	vt.	to make food, drink, etc. go down your throat into your stomach 吞下；咽下
targeted	/ˈtɑːgɪtɪd/	adj.	directed; oriented 定向的
therapy	/ˈθerəpi/	n.	the treatment of a physical problem or an illness 治疗；疗法
therapist	/ˈθerəpɪst/	n.	a specialist who treats a particular type of illness or problem, or who uses a particular type of treatment（某治疗法的）治疗专家
utensil	/juːˈtensl/	n.	a tool that is used in the house 用具；器皿

Proper names

active ROM	主动关节活动度
ankle pump	踝泵
cardiac events	心脏事件
Cognitive Rehabilitation	认知康复
Occupational Therapy	职业疗法
passive ROM	被动关节活动度
Physical Therapy	物理疗法
respiratory distress	呼吸窘迫
Respiratory Therapy	呼吸疗法
Speech Therapy	语言障碍矫正；言语治疗
Vocational Rehabilitation	职业康复

Unit 8　Community Care

accessible	/əkˈsesəbl/	adj.	capable of being reached 可到达的；可接近的
cardiologist	/ˌkɑːrdiˈɑːlədʒɪst/	n.	a doctor who specializes in cardiology 心脏病医生；心脏病学家
condom	/ˈkɑːndəm/	n.	a sheath commonly of rubber worn over the penis（as to prevent conception or venereal infection during coitus）避孕套
discipline	/ˈdɪsəplɪn/	n.	a field of study 学科
eliminate	/ɪˈlɪmɪneɪt/	vt.	to put an end to or get rid of 排除；清除；消除
implementation	/ˌɪmpləmɛnˈteɪʃən/	n.	the process of making something active or effective 完成；履行；执行
incorporate	/ɪnˈkɔːrpəreɪt/	v.	to blend or combine thoroughly 将…包括在内；包含；吸收；使并入
internist	/ɪnˈtɜːrnɪst/	n.	a specialist in internal medicine 内科医生
nutrient	/ˈnuːtriənt/	n.	a substance or ingredient that promotes growth, provides energy, and maintains life 营养素；营养物
obesity	/oʊˈbisəti/	n.	a condition characterized by the excessive accumulation and storage of fat in the body 肥胖症
occurrence	/əˈkɜːrəns/	n.	the action or fact of happening or occurring —often used with of 发生的事情；存在的事物；发生；出现；存在
re – emerging	/ˌriːɪˈmɜːrdʒɪŋ/	adj.	formed or prominentagain 再出现的
rheumatologist	/ruməˈtɒlədʒɪst/	n.	Specialist in conditions and diseases of the muscles and skeletal system, especially those affecting the joints. 风湿病学家；风湿病医生；风湿病专家
respiratory	/ˈrespərətɔːri/	adj.	a single complete act of breathing 呼吸的
socioeconomic	/ˌsəʊsɪəʊˌɛkəˈnɒmɪk/	adj.	relating to, or involving a combination of social and economic factors 社会经济的
urologist	/jʊrˈɒlədʒɪst/	n.	a physician who specializes in the urinary or urogenital tract 泌尿科医生
vulnerable	/ˈvʌlnərəbl/	adj.	capable of being physically or emotionally wounded（身体上或感情上）脆弱的，易受…伤害的
Proper names			
administer immunizations			接种疫苗
chronic condition			慢性状况；
cough syrup			咳嗽糖浆

dispense medications	配药
infectious and sexually transmitted diseases	传染病和性传播疾病
poor nutrition	营养不良
rheumatic plaster	风湿膏
substance abuse	药物滥用
teen pregnancy	未成年怀孕

Unit 9　Hospice Care

acronym	/ˈækrənɪm/	n.	a word formed from the initial letters of the several words in the name 首字母缩略词
acupuncture	/ˈækjupʌŋktʃə/	n.	a Chinese method of treating pain and illness using special thin needles which are pushed into the skin inparticular parts of the body 针刺疗法
adjuvant	/ˈædʒʊvənt/	n.	辅药，佐药，佐剂
advanced	/ədˈvɑːnst/	adj.	Something that is at an advanced stage or level is at a late stage of development. 晚期的；后期的
alleviate	/əˈliːvieɪ/	vt.	provide physical relief, as from pain 减轻；缓和；缓解
analgesic	/ˌænəlˈdʒiːzɪk/	n.	a medicine used to relieve pain 止痛药；镇痛剂
anxiety	/æŋˈzaɪəti/	n.	the state of feeling nervous or worried that sth. bad is going to happen 焦虑；忧虑
bedsore	/ˈbedsɔː(r)/	n.	a painful and sometimes infected place on aperson's skin, caused by lying in bed for a long time 褥疮
chemotherapy	/ˌkiːməʊˈθerəpi/	n.	the treatment of disease, especially cancer, with the use of chemical substances 化学疗法，化疗
clergy	/ˈklɜːrdʒi/	n.	（统称）圣职人员，神职人员
coma	/ˈkəʊmə/	n.	a deep unconsciousstate, usually lasting a long time and caused by serious illness or injury 昏迷
counselor	/ˈkaʊns(ə)lə/	n.	someone who gives advice about problems 顾问
denial	/dɪˈnaɪəl/	n.	a refusal to accept that sth. unpleasant or painful is true 否认（令人不快、痛苦的事）
dietitian	/ˌdaɪəˈtɪʃn/	n.	饮食学家；营养学家
digestible	/daɪˈdʒestəbl/	adj.	easy to digest; pleasant to eat 易消化的；口感好的
dignity	/ˈdɪgnəti/	n.	formality in bearing and appearance 尊严；尊贵

dyspnea	/dɪspˈniːə/	n.	difficult or labored respiration 呼吸困难
empathy	/ˈempəθi/	n.	theability to understand another person's feelings, experience, etc. 同感；同情；共鸣
fatigue	/fəˈtiːg/	n.	a feeling of being extremely tired, usually because of hard work or exercise 疲劳；劳累
fragility	/frəˈdʒɪlɪti/	n.	lack of physical strength 脆弱；虚弱
hospice	/ˈhɒspɪs/	n.	a hospital for people who are dying 临终安养院
immortal	/ɪˈmɔːtl/	n.	神；永生不灭者
indigestion	/ˌɪndɪˈdʒestʃən/	n.	pain caused by difficulty in digesting food 消化不良（症）
jargon	/ˈdʒɑːgən/	n.	行话；行业术语
massage	/ˈmæsɑːʒ/	n.	the action of rubbing andpressing a person'sbody with the hands to reduce pain in themuscles and joints 按摩
mnemonic	/nɪˈmɒnɪk/	n.	a word, sentence, poem, etc. that helps you to remember sth. 帮助记忆的词句（或诗歌等）；助记符号
numb	/nʌm/	adj.	unable to feel, think or react in the normal way 麻木的；迟钝的；呆滞的
option	/ˈɒpʃn/	n.	the act of choosing or selecting 选择；选择权
palliation	/ˌpæliˈeɪʃən/	n.	easing the severity of a pain or a disease without removing the cause （痛苦的）减轻；缓和
pancreatic	/ˌpæŋkriˈætɪk/	adj.	of or involving the pancreas 胰（腺）的
paradise	/ˈpærədaɪs/	n.	(in some religions) a perfect place where people are said to go when they die（某些宗教所指的）天堂，天国
perception	/pəˈsepʃn/	n.	the ability to understand the true nature of sth. 悟性，看法，见解
protocol	/ˈprəʊtəkɒl/	n.	a plan for performing a scientificexperiment or medical treatment 科学实验计划；医疗方案
recurrence	/rɪˈkʌrəns/	n.	happening again 复发
source	/sɔːs/	n.	a place, person or thing that you get sth. from 来源；出处
suicidal	/ˌsuːɪˈsaɪdl/	adj.	想自杀的；有自杀倾向的
therapist	/ˈθerəpɪst/	n.	a specialist who treats aparticular type of illness or problem, or who uses a particular type of treatment （某治疗法的）治疗专家
tumor	/tjuːmə(r)/	n.	肿瘤

Proper names	
acupuncture and moxibustion	针灸
religious faith	宗教信仰
medical term	医学术语
liver transplant	肝移植
tube feeding	管饲法
amyotrophic lateral sclerosis	肌萎缩侧索硬化（ALS）
occupational therapist	职业治疗师（利用特定的技能训练帮助病患者或受伤者恢复健康）
swallowing disorder	吞咽障碍
clan custom	宗族习俗

Answer Key

Unit 1　Admitting Patients

Warm – up Exercises

A. ID card　B. Medical insurance card　C. Outpatient medical record

Reading

■ Task 1

1. j　2. i　3. h　4. g　5. f　6. e　7. d　8. c　9. b　10. a

■ Task 2

1. secure　2. sit on　3. be performed　4. past hospitalizations and surgeries　5. is located

■ Task 3

1. One form may be a detailed medical and medication history. Another form is called a living will and clearly tells which specific resuscitation efforts the person does or does not want to have performed on them in order to save or extend their life.

2. Yes, I do.

Receive the patient into the system in such a manner that he/she feels welcome and secure while comfort, safety, biopsychosocial, cultural, financial and spiritual needs are addressed.

Listening and Speaking

Activity 1　welcoming a patient on admission

■ Task 1

1. e　2. a　3. b　4. c　5. d　6. h　7. g　8. f　9. j　10. i

■ Task 2

A：Name　B：Sex　C：Date of Birth　E：Address　D：Tel　F：Allergic History

■ Task 3

1. bothering　2. registration　3. fourth floor　4. corridor　5. exception

■ Task 4

1. have a headache　2. have a fever　3. have muscle soreness　4. feel dizzy　5. the day before yesterday

6. on business　7. first　8. medical department

Activity 2　Going through the Admission Procedure

■ Task 1

1. e　2. b　3. c　4. d　5. a

■ Task 2

1. taking care of　2. admission procedure　3. appointment card　4. name　5. date of birth

6. May 7th, 1965

■ Task 3

1. He lives at No. 45 Shandong Road, Jinzhou.

2. He had a slipped disc two years ago.

3. Penicillin.

4. In order to fill in the admission form.

■ Task 4

1. 120/80 mmHg   2. 50 beats/m   3. 36.5℃   4. 18 breaths/m

Activity 3   Taking Patients to the Ward

■ Task 1

A. ward room   B. bed number   C. bracelet   D. call button   E. curtain

■ Task 2

1. ECG examination   2. chest X – ray   3. third   4. coronary heart

■ Task 3

1. F   2. F   3. F   4. T   5. T

■ Task 4

1. Six.

2. He was not used to being in the hospital.

3. Not good. It will help him recover more quickly.

4. He feels dizzy all the time. The nurse will insert the oxygen cannula.

Writing

John Smith isa 18 years old boy. He was admitted in the hospital on September 7th. He complained that he had difficulty in breathing and vomited once every hour. He suffered from abdominal pain and diarrhea.

The physical examination shows that the boy is running a high temperature of 40℃. His pulse is 94 times per minute, respiratory rate is 20 minutes per minute and blood pressure is 123/80mmHg.

According to the history and assessment, the boy is likely to be under the condition of dehydration. Major nursing instructions for him are given as follow. The boy should be encouraged to have much fluid and daily fluid intake of 2500 ml. He should have a rest on bed for 2 days.

Unit 2   Administering Medications

Warm – up Exercises

A – tablet   B – inhaler   C – liquid   D – capsule   E – topicalmedicine   F – patch   G – suppository
H – drop   I – injection

Tablets are usually taken orally but can be administered sublingually, buccally, rectally, or intravaginally.

Inhalers are dispersed via an aerosol spray, mist, or powder that patients inhale into their airways.

Liquids are usually taken orally. Liquid medicines include liquids, solutions, syrups, and mixtures and are commonly used in patients with difficulty swallowing drugs.

Capsules usually are swallowed whole with water, milk, food, or juice. Some work best on an empty stomach.

Topical medicines are creams, lotions or ointments applied directly onto the skin.

Patches are applied directly to the skin.

The suppository is inserted into the rectum.

Drops tend to be used for eye, ear, or nose.

Injections are normally administered intradermally, subcutaneously, intravenously, and intramuscularly.

Reading

■ **Task 1**

1. j 2. a 3. h 4. f 5. b 6. c 7. g 8. d 9. e 10. i

■ **Task 2**

1. dosage 2. allergy 3. one 4. antidotes 5. respiratory

■ **Task 3**

1. Yes, medication safety and taking precautionary steps are extremely important to prevent adverse reactions, overdoses and death.

2. In order to avoid compromising patient safety, nurses should refer to and adhere to the principles of drug administration. Nurses are responsible for the administration of medicines. Therefore, they must ensure that they are careful at all times and that patient safety is central to this process.

Listening and Speaking

Activity 1 Identifying Prescription

■ **Task 1**

1. d 2. a 3. b 4. c 5. e 6. k 7. h 8. f 9. g 10. i 11. j 12. l 13. o 14. m 15. n 16. p

■ **Task 2**

Line A	It is the preprinted name of the physician or group of physicians, the address, and phone number.
Line B	It includes the patient's name, address, date of the prescription, and the patient's age if the patient is a child.
Line C	It is the superscription or the symbol, meaning "recipe" or "take thou", from Latin.
Line D	It includes the name of the medication, its strength, and the quantity of drugs to be dispensed.
Line E	It is the "Sig", or "signa", giving directions for taking the medication.
Line F	It tells the pharmacist the drug form, as well as how the medication is be taken.
Line G	It tells the physician's signature.
Line H	It tells the number of allowed refills.
Line I	If the prescription is for a controlled medication, the physician must place his or her U. S. Drug Enforcement Administration (DEA) number either under or beside the signa.

■ **Task 3**

1. 5ml; two times; 10 2. mouth 3. 100ml; doctor 4. brand

■ **Task 4**

1. Lucas 2. 9/18/2013 3. Boni Avenue, Machester City 4. 54 5. 500 6. capsule 7. 3 8. None

Activity 2 Doing a Medication Check

■ **Task 1**

1. b 2. d 3. e 4. a 5. c

■ **Task 2**

1. have you got a minute

2. occupied with something

3. available

4. Are you free at the moment

5. I'm up to my eyeballs

6. Are you busy at the moment

7. treating room

■ **Task 3**

1. Humulin N insulin

2. Insulin is designed to be taken before eating to help control blood sugar. If a patient waits too long to eat, his blood sugar can actually end up getting too low which is dangerous to a patient.

3. The order on the MAR contains the patient's name, the drug name, the drug dosage, administration method and time; the medication label contains the drug name, dosage, expire date.

4. They both have to sign their names in the drug book.

5. They do the double check for the medication. They communicate with each other clearly and read the medication record correctly.

■ **Task 4**

1. c　2. d　3. a　4. e　5. b　6. f　7. g

Activity 3　Administering Medications

■ **Task 1**

A: Injection: It is a way of administering a sterile liquid form of medication into tissues of the body beneath the skin, usually using a sharp, hollow needle or tube.

B: Oral administration: It is a route of administration where a substance is taken through the mouth.

C: Topical medication administration: Topical route of drug administration commonly refers to the application of medication to the skin's surface. Topical medication includes creams, foams, gels, lotions, and ointments.

D: Ear drops medication administration: The nurses carefully place drops into the ear canal.

E: Rectal drug administration: The nurses slowly insert the lubricated suppository into the rectum.

F: Inhalation: Inhalation is the route by which the medication is breathed directly into the pathway to the lungs. This route is typically used for direct administration to the organ desired, the lungs, and it is used in pediatric patients for easier medication delivery.

■ **Task 2**

1. Insulin

2. The nurse will administer the drug subcutaneously. Three times a day and 30 minutes before breakfast, lunch and dinner.

3. Yes, they do. They verify medication order and make sure it is complete, check the patient's medical record for an allergy, prepare medication for one patient at a time, educate patients about their medication and double – check the medicine and patients.

■ **Task 3**

4　3　2　7　5　6　1　8

▉ Task 4

1. eye infection   2. eye drops   3. two drops per time   4. Metamucil   5. oral

6. three times per day at mealtime   7. cold   8. tablet   9. every six hours

Writing

Mr. Xin Yang is a 45 – year – old who was diagnosed with Type 2 diabetes at 30 years old. His doctor prescribed Humulin N insulin to him to control his blood sugar level. The drug should be administered 115 units via subcutaneous injection, three times a day, and 30 minutes before each meal. This morning, Xin Yang was administered Humulin N insulin 115 units in the abdomen at 7：30 am by nurse Susan. Both Susan and Joan did the crosscheck about the medication label and MAR. After the injection, Mr. Yang didn't have any discomfort. And the breakfast was served at 7：50 am.

Unit 3   Preventing Cross Infection

Warm – up Exercises

1. There are many risk factors for infection such as skin and mucous membrane damage, needle stick injury or sharp instrument injury, needle stick injury, hand pollution, air pollution.

2. There are many ways to prevent infection. For example, wash your hands well; cover a cough; wash and bandage all cuts; do not pick at healing wounds or blemishes or squeeze pimples; don't share dishes, glasses, or eating utensils. Avoid direct contact with napkins, tissues, handkerchiefs, or similar items used by others.

3. Under clean running water (warm or cold), wet your hands.

Turn off the water (think of the environment and save water!).

Apply soap to your hands. Soap can be liquid, bar or powder.

Lather the soap and rub your hands together for more than 20 seconds, being sure to scrub all surfaces, including backs of hands, wrists, between fingers, and under fingernails.

Turnthe water back on and rinse hands well.

Turnthe water off using the back of your hand or a towel.

Dry your hands with an air dryer while rubbing hands together, or use a towel.

Reading

▉ Task 1

1. h   2. g   3. c   4. a   5. i   6. b   7. d   8. e   9. j   10. f

▉ Task 2

1. self – protection   2. disinfection   3. infection   4. simultaneously   5. hygiene

▉ Task 3

1. Yes, infection control is important. It can ensure that patients have access to safe medical and health services.

2. Source of infectious microorganisms, susceptible persons, and means of transmission.

Listening and Speaking

Activity 1   Preventing Cross Infection among Medical Staff

▉ Task 1

1. c   2. e   3. a   4. b   5. d   6. j   7. g   8. i   9. h   10. f

■ **Task 2**

1. infectious disease   2. personal protection   3. overemphasize   4. droplets   5. syringe

■ **Task 3**

1. c   2. g   3. e   4. f   5. a   6. b   7. d

■ **Task 4**

1. isolation gown   2. clean   3. stretch   4. parallel   5. Tie

■ **Task 5**

1. d   2. a   3. c   4. b   5. e

Activity 2   Doing aNucleic Acid Test

■ **Task 1**

1. e   2. a   3. b   4. c   5. d   6. h   7. j   8. f   9. i   10. g

■ **Task 2**

1. running   2. sore   3. inflamed   4. mercury thermometer   5. nucleic

■ **Task 3**

1. It is a technique used to detect and identify whether the coronavirus infects you.

2. It enables the nasal passage become more accessible.

3. Firstly, take off the mask; secondly, blow the nose; thirdly, tilt the head back; fourthly, close the eyes; fifthly, insert a swab into the nose; lastly, put on the mask again.

■ **Task 4**

1. c   2. b   3. a   4. e   5. d   6. f

Activity 3   Informing the Interventions about Preventing Cross Infections

■ **Task 1**

A: 3M mask

B: Isolation gown

C: Goggles

D: Handheld thermometer

E: Sterile cap

F: Mercury thermometer

■ **Task 2**

1. infectious   2. high – risk   3. escort   4. sterile   5. mask   6. recovery

■ **Task 3**

1. No, it isn't. The hospital is a high – risk area where people gather.

2. No, it is not allowed to pay a visit to infectious patients.

3. The visitors should wear a sterile isolation gown and isolation shoes, wear a mask, and wash hands with sterile water after the visit.

■ **Task 4**

1. community   2. sanitizer   3. touch   4. feet   5. instructions   6. virus

■ **Task 5**

Writing

1. Control the sources of infection and cut off the channels of transmission.

2. Make every possible effort to curb the spread of the disease.

3. Build stringent lines of defense across society.

4. Prevent the coronavirus from spreading within the city/region or beyond.

5. Drug and vaccine development.

Unit 4　Preparing Patients for Radiology

Warm – up Exercises

A – Angiogram　B – CT – scan　C – Mammogram　D – MRI　E – Ultrasound　F – X – ray

Angiography is a kind of interventional detection method, which injects the contrast agent into the blood vessel. Because X – ray can not penetrate the contrast agent, angiography is to use this property, through the X – ray image of the contrast agent to diagnose vascular lesions.

CT examination is mainly aimed at scanning the human brain. CT examination generally includes plain CT, enhanced CT and cisternography CT.

Ina mammogram, the structure of the breast is shown in black and white.

Magnetic resonance imaging (MRI) has been used to diagnose various systems of the whole body. The best effect is the brain, and its spinal cord, heart and blood vessels, joint bone, soft tissue, and pelvic cavity.

B ultrasound is the use of ultrasound and human organs and tissues acoustic interaction, the formation of graphics, curves, etc., to diagnose diseases.

X – ray imaging is to show different tissues of the human body at different levels.

Reading

■ **Task 1**

1. e　2. f　3. a　4. d　5. b　6. c

■ **Task 2**

1. X – ray; CT　2. density; whiter　3. Contrast agents　4. ultrasonography　5. MRI

■ **Task 3**

1. Yes, imaging tests in hospital isessential. It is because imaging tests provide a picture of the body's interior—of the whole body or part of it. Imaging helps doctors diagnose a disorder, determine how severe the disorder is, and monitor people after the condition is diagnosed.

2. It is because there will be radiation in some imaging examinations, such as X – ray, CT, etc.

Listening and Speaking

Activity 1　Getting CT Scan Consent for IV Contrast Injection

■ **Task 1**

1. g　2. a　3. b　4. d　5. e　6. c　7. f

■ **Task 2**

1. Enhanced CT scan

2. The medical staff should assess the patients' allergic history, medical history, maternal history and drug history.

3. Informed consent creates trust between doctor and patient by ensuring good understanding. It also reduces the risk for both patient and doctor.

■ **Task 3**

1. chest tightness; fever   2. allergic   3. suffering from   4. make sure   5. precautions; observe

■ **Task 4**

1. There will be some discomfort and allergic reactions, such as chest tightness, nausea, fever, rash, etc.

2. Firstly, after the examination, sit for 30 minutes and observe whether there is any discomfort. Secondly, after the examination, drink more water, which can accelerate the discharge of contrast medium.

3. Yes, he has heart disease.

■ **Task 5**

Practice dialogue with each other.

Activity 2   Preparing a Patient for CT Scan

■ **Task 1**

1—B   2—A   3—C

■ **Task 2**

(1) chest CT examination   (2) metal items   (3) CT images   (4) breath holding

(5) gown   (6) wheelchair

■ **Task 3**

1. Chest CT – scan

2. Take off metal items, practice breath holding, put on special gown.

3. About an hour

■ **Task 4**

9 – 3 – 8 – 10 – 4 – 5 – 6 – 7 – 1 – 2

■ **Task 5**

Practice dialogue with each other.

Activity 3   Preparing a Patient for Chest X – ray

■ **Task 1**

1. c   2. b   3. e   4. a   5. d   6. f

■ **Task 2**

1. intradermal test   2. penicillin   3. 0. 1 ml   4. 15 minutes   5. Oral test

■ **Task 3**

5 – 2 – 6 – 4 – 1 – 3

■ **Task 4**

1. intradermal   2. disinfect   3. massage   4. itchy; bump

■ **Task 5**

Practice dialogue with each other.

Writing

This is not the only answer, just for reference. Students can query the latest authoritative research results from websites such as CNKI and PubMed.

Medical imaging examination is an important part of physical examination. It can use the most advanced instruments and equipment to achieve early detection, early diagnosis and early treatment. Therefore, I agree to perform imagingexamination. Various examinations will have certain risks due to the patient's personal physical condition, time, condition, machine, etc. , but with the continuous development and maturity of medical technology, try to minimize the incidence of various risks. At present, some studies show that CT examination shows that DNA exposed to radiation has the potential risk of change, but the incidence is not high.

Unit 5　Caring for Operative Patients

Warm – up Exercises

A – PCA pump　B – Intravenous indwelling needle　C – Drainage catheter　D – Endotracheal cannula
E – Surgical incision dressing　F – Antibiotics　G – Monitor　H – Ventilator　I – Indwelling urinary catheter

Indwelling urinary catheter is inserted into the urinary bladder for therapeutic or diagnostic purposes and ·temporarily retained in the bladder to drain urine.

Drainage catheter is placed at the surgical incision during the operation. Blood and body fluids can be discharged from the body through the catheter to promote the healing of the incision, and at the same time, it is convenient to observe the color, shape and amount of the drainage fluid.

Antibiotics are mainly used to treat various bacterial infections or pathogenic microbial infections. It can be divided into natural antibiotics, semi – synthetic antibiotics and fully synthetic antibiotics.

Endotracheal cannula is a special artificial airway that can be inserted directly into the trachea through the glottis via the mouth or the nose to maintain the airway smoothness, perform sputum suction, or connect to a ventilator for assisted ventilation.

Patient Controlled Analgesic (PCA) pump is a device that allows patients to administer pre – set doses of pain medications according to their pain conditions through computer control or mechanical principles.

Ventilator is a device that can replace, control or change a person's normal physiological breathing, increase lung ventilation, improve respiratory function, reduce respiratory work consumption, and save heart reserve capacity.

Monitor is a device used to monitor the vital signs of patients, including heart rate, blood pressure, respiration, oxygen saturation, etc.

Surgical incision dressing is a material used to bandage wounds and cover sores, wounds or other damages.

Intravenous indwelling needle is consists of a flexible catheter that can be placed in a blood vessel and a stainless steel puncture guide needle core. It can reduce the pain and vascular damage caused by repeated punctures and keep the venous passage open.

Reading

■■ **Task 1**

1. e　2. g　3. a　4. d　5. j　6. b　7. i　8. c　9. f　10. h

■■ **Task 2**

1. Enhanced recovery nursing is on the basis of evidence – based nursing, based on holistic nursing, and taking nursing intervention as measures to optimize and integrate the latest nursing concepts, establish clinical nursing procedures, implement clinical nursing pathways, and achieve the purpose of accelerating rehabilitation.

2. I. Preoperative preparation

(1) Preoperative education

(2) Screening and treatment of malnutrition

（3）Fasting and oral carbohydrates

（4）Preventive antithrombotic treatment

（5）Pulmonary rehabilitation exercise

II. Surgery day：（1）Check the patient's identity and information.

（2）Do the handover work of preoperative and postoperative.

III. Post–operative care：（1）Observes the patient's vital signs and condition changes.

（2）Follows the doctor's instructions to use drugs.

■ Task 3

1. preoperative education, antibacterial drugs, blood pressure, blood sugar control.

2. 6, 2.

3. 400, 12.5, 2.

4. the surgeon, anesthesiologist, operating room nurse.

Listening and Speaking

Activity 1Doing a Preoperative Checks

■ Task 1

1. e 2. d 3. f 4. j 5. i 6. c 7. a 8. h 9. b 10. g

■ Task 2

1. F 2. F 3. F 4. F 5. T 6. F

■ Task 3

1. d 2. c 3. a 4. b 5. e

■ Task 4

1. total knee arthroplasty of right knee; 8：00

2. prepare it well; get through; smoothly

3. quit; taking deep breathing; effective cough

4. Gastrointestinal; gastric contents reflux; aspiration

5. Patient's gown; denture, glasses and jewelry; valuables

Activity 2 Filling aPreoperative Checklist

■ Task 1

1 – b　2 – c　3 – d　4 – e　5 – a　6 – f

■ Task 2

General condition of the patient	
Hospitalnumber：<u>6523241</u> Bed number：<u>13</u> Name：<u>John Steward</u>　Age：<u>65</u> Gender：<u>male</u> Department：　<u>Orthopedics</u>	Preoperative diagnosis：<u>osteoarthritis of both knees</u> Name of proposed operation：<u>Total knee arthroplasty of right knee</u> Planned operation time：　<u>8am on Sep 17th</u>

Operation history：Yes No √	
Past history： ___Hypertension___	
Allergy history： No √ Yes	
Blood type： A√ B AB O RH（ + √ – ）	
Blood – borne diseases：No √ Yes	
Vein condition：Filled √ generally hard not touchable	
Physical activity：free √ obstacles	
Skin condition：intact √ damaged： _____	
Nutritional status：good √ average poor	

■ Task 3

1. Temp's thirty – six seven, pulse is 78. Resps are 18 breaths a minute. BP is one hundred and thirty – five over eighty – four. Body weight is 84.5 kilos.

2. He had dinner at around 18：00 last night, and haven't eaten anything since. The last time he drank water was about half an hour ago, around 5：30 this morning.

3. She checked the back of the left hand and the surgical site.

■ Task 4

ABCF

Activity 3   Caring for aPatient in Recovery Room

■ Task 1

1 – d 2 – b 3 – a 4 – c

■ Task 2

☑ body temperature	☑ surgical incision dressing
☑ blood pressure	☑ the fixation and drainage of the patient's drainage tube
☑ respiratory rate and tidal volume	☐ thirsty
☑ consciousness	☑ IV infusion

■ Task 3

1. Observe whether the patient opens his eyes spontaneously. If no, call the patient's name, or tap the patient's shoulder to see if the patient has an eye – opening response and eye contact.

2. Assess the patient's motor response following commands.

3. Ask simple questions to see whether the patient could understand.

■ Task 4

1. C 2. D 3. A 4. E 5. B

Writing

John Steward, hospitalization number 6523241, male, 65 – year – old, will accept total knee arthroplasty of right knee today. He has been quitting smoke for one month and already been told the way of effective cough training after operation. He has fasted more than 8 hours from diet and 2 hours from water. Last night he had no sleep disorder. Vital signs taken this morning are normal. He has changed the patient's uniform and had no dentures, jewelry, glasses and other personal belongings with him. The intravenous infusion channel is on the back of the left hand, there is no tube on the body, the surgical site has been marked, the skin is intact, and there is no high risk of pressure sores.

Unit 6   Discharging Patients

Warm – up Exercises

A. Recheck   B. Sports and exercise   C. Medication   D. Living habits   E. Discharge summary   F. Diet

Reading

▮▮ Task 1

1. d   2. e   3. i   4. c   5. b   6. h   7. g   8. j   9. f   10. a

▮▮ Task 2

1. Discharge   2. the discharge nurse   3. follow – up appointments   4. Providers   5. 14 – 30 days

▮▮ Task 3

1. The patients must have a clear understanding of their medical conditions and what must be done to continue care as an outpatient, must receive an explanation of potential warning signs and symptoms that could arise, should be provided with a 24 – hour phone number for emergencies, should have the name of the provider responsible for their care after discharge.

2. All instructions for care at home, including medications, diet, therapy, and follow – up appointments.

Listening and Speaking

Activity 1   Giving instructions to patients – 1 (Diet and Medication)

▮▮ Task 1

1. i   2. h   3. g   4. j   5. a   6. c   7. e   8. b   9. f   10. d

▮▮ Task 2

A: Patient Name   B: Discharge Date   C: Attending Physician   E: Discharge Diagnosis

D: Attending Diagnosis   F: Discharge Instructions

▮▮ Task 3

1. good; tomorrow   2. a discharge certificate   3. three   4. regularly; worsens

▮▮ Task 4

1. low – salt   2. spicy   3. quantitative   4. mental stress   5. smoking   6. stimulate the incision

7. two tablets   8. chest pain

Activity 2   Giving instructions to patients – 2 (Exercise, Recheck and Discharge Procedure)

▮▮ Task 1

1. c   2. e   3. a   4. b   5. f   6. d

▮▮ Task 2

1. When can I be discharged

2. you were well recovered

3. be discharged

4. I have been in the hospital for three weeks

5. for a long time

■ Task 3

1. It contains the dosage of drugs and precautions.

2. After a week, Mr. King can start doing some light exercise.

3. Yes. Because they can improve muscle oxygen transport capacity and improve cardiopulmonary function.

4. Mr. King is going to take the bill at the doctor's office. He can pay it in cash or check.

5. Yes. Mr. King needs to go back to the hospital for a checkup in two weeks.

■ Task 4

1. d　2. a, b, f, i　3. c, g　4. e, h

Activity 3　Making a referral of a patient

■ Task 1

a, b, c, d, e, g, i, j

■ Task 2

1. Because Susan needs to refer her patient, Selena, to the District Care Service Center for some district care services.

2. She had a stroke about a month ago.

3. She is hemiplegic in the right side of her body. She is inarticulate and has difficulty swallowing. She can't move easily. She can't take a bath by herself and can't stand steadily.

4. Her GP is Dr. Harrison.

5. She can eat some soft food that is easy to digest. About 50 mg.

■ Task 3

1. F　2. T　3. F　4. F　5. T

■ Task 4

1. Selena　2. 81　3. 7083926　4. 15966304528　5. Harrison　6. stroke　7. can't move easily

8. can't take a bath　9. can't stand steadily　10. soft food

Writing

Date：21/09/2020

To：District Nursing Nurse,

District Nursing Service Center, 124 High Street, Dongshan District.

Subject：referral of patient's care to District Nursing Service Center

Dear Sir/Madam,

I am writing with regards to the referral of Mrs. Selena, aged 81, will be discharged tomorrow. She is inarticulate and has difficulty swallowing. She can't move easily and can't take a bath by herself. She can't stand steadily and has to use a walking frame. Her daughter, Lucy, usually takes care of her. And her GP is Dr. Harrison.

The patient needs some daily life and food care. She still needs to eat some soft food that is easy to digest these days. She was asked to eat soft food that was easy to digest. About 50 milligrams each meal.

Do contact me if you require any clarifications of the case.

Thank you.

Yours sincerely,

Susan

Unit 7　Facilitating Patients' Rehabilitation

Warm – up Exercises

A – neck extension　　B – shoulder abduction　　C – shoulder adduction　　D – knee bend　　E – wrist stretch

F – ankle pump　　G – ankle rotation　　H – toe raise　　I – elbow flexion

Susan is supposed to choose A, D, F and G.

Reading

■ **Task 1**

1. d　2. f　3. a　4. g　5. i　6. j　7. c　8. e　9. b　10. h

■ **Task 2**

1. designed　2. focuses on　3. geared towards　4. vary　5. appropriate

■ **Task 3**

1. Physical therapy works to improve movement dysfunction. Occupational therapy focuses on restoring an individual's ability to perform necessary daily activities.

2. When multiple types of therapy are needed to aid an individual in recovery and rehabilitation or close medical supervision is necessary, seeking services in an inpatient facility is generally recommended as the safest and most efficient means of treatment.

Listening and Speaking

Activity 1　Assessing Activities of Daily Living (ADLs)

■ **Task 1**

A. walking stick　　B. urinal bottle　　C. walking frame　　D. commode　　E. shower chair　　F. bedpan

■ **Task 2**

ADLs	1. **Karl**	2. **Ellen**	3. **Selina**
washing	*independent*	*dependent*	
dressing		*dependent*	*independent*
grooming	*dependent*		
oral hygiene			*independent*

■ **Task 3**

1. Karl suffers from early dementia.

2. He needs assistance with simple tasks, such as shaving, washing, and eating.

3. Nurse Susanis very impolite and lacks empathy.

4. She thinks she is very busy and not paid enough to clean up.

5. She is supposed to bemore friendly, understanding and respectful for her patients.

▰ Task 4

	no empathy	a little empathy	a lot of empathy
Nurse 1		✓	
Nurse 2	✓		
Nurse 3			✓

Activity 2　Measuring aPatient's Range of Motion（ROM）

▰ Task 1

A. extension　B. abduction　C. flexion　D. adduction　E. rotation

▰ Task 2

1. He's a little tired this morning.

2. The old exercises are a little too easy.

3. He starts with the right leg.

4. It's tough at first, but he can feel getting stronger.

▰ Task 3

1. immobilized　2. active ROM　3. mobile　4. discomfort　5. limited to　6. passive ROM

▰ Task 4

Flow sheet – ROM（range of motion exercises）		
Patient：Bill Smith　　**Room No.**：Bed 34　　**Date**：18/06/2021　　**Time**：9 a. m.		
Movement	Result	Comments
R shoulder flexion	1. ✓	WNL
R shoulder rotation	2. ✓	WNL
R elbow extension	3. ✓	7. WNL withno pain
R elbow flexion	4. ✓	8. WNL withsome pain
L shoulder flexion	5. ✓	9. limited to 120°
L shoulder extension	6. X	10. not able to do
Nurse's initials	GPR	

Activity 3　SettingGoals and Giving Encouragement

▰ Task 1

1. B　2. A.　3. C

▰ Task 2

1. What's your long – term goal?

2. What do you want to do today?

3. What can you do?

4. For today our goal is three sets of ten on each arm.

5. Can you do that?

6. Can you do this exercise three times a day?

■ **Task 3**

2. 4. 8

■ **Task 4**

1. F   2. T   3. T   4. F   5. T

Writing

Bill Smith is a 27 – year – old man. He suffered from a road accident on July 20th, 2021. He was conscious but tired with nausea. There was bruising and swelling on his left shoulder. The ROM assessment indicated that his limit was 100 degrees with significant discomfort. His left leg was immobilized, while other joints were fully mobile fortunately. Before this accident, Mr. Smith's health status was excellent, so he was unwilling to perform ROM. Currently, we intend to plan ROM exercises for him. For the 1st stage, we will begin with passive ROM exercises two times a day. We will move his joint through the range of motion with no effort from him. For the 2nd stage, we have to teach Mr. Smith to perform active ROM three times a day. At that moment, he will be expected to perform the exercise to move the joint without any assistance to the muscles surrounding the joint, which would be the most appropriate for the patient's recovery.

Unit 8   Community Care

Warm – up Exercises

A Aging population

B Community – based elderly care

C Pension insurance

D Delay retirement

E To pay filial respects for one's parents

F Empty nest old

Reading

■ **Task 1**

1. c   2. a   3. g   4. d   5. b   6. j   7. i   8. h   9. e   10. f

■ **Task 2**

1. These caregivers

2. Community health nursing

3. condoms and pregnancy tests.

4. provide treatment to patients.

5. community centers, government health agencies

■ **Task 3**

1. The goal of community health nursing is to promote, protect and preserve the health of the public.

2. Because they can travel to remote places and isolated areas of a city.

Listening and Speaking

Activity 1   Talking about Nutrition for the Elderly

■ **Task 1**

1. b   2. c   3. a   4. g   5. d   6. e   7. j   8. f   9. h   10. i

■ **Task 2**

1. b   2. d   3. e   4. a   5. c   6. f   7. h   8. g

■ **Task 3**

1. T   2. T   3. F   4. F   5. T

■ **Task 4**

balanceddiet；routine life；regular physical exercises；nutrition

■ **Task 5**

Reference answer：

Patient：Good morning.

Nurse：Good morning. What can I help you?

Patient：I feel less and less appetite recently.

Nurse：Have you had a physical examination?

Patient：I went to the hospital for examination. The doctor said there was nothing wrong except that the blood pressure was a little high. What should I do to improve my appetite

Nurse：You should eat more digestible food and take part in more exercise.

Patient：What foods can help digestion?

Nurse：Eat more foods rich in crude fiber such as sweet potato，vegetable or add some dietary fiber supplements. If you have constipation，eating more crude fiber can also improve it.

Patient：Yes，I have the constipation. Can I smoke?

Nurse：Smoking is harmful to anyone's health. Better give it up.

Patient：Thanks very much. That's very helpful.

Nurse：You are welcome.

Activity 2　Applying Home Medication Management for Seniors

■ **Task 1**

1. b   2. a   3. d   4. c   5. e

■ **Task 2**

1. The patient has a terrible cold.

2. No，he doesn't.

3. No，he can't.

4. The nurse recommended vitamin C effervescent tablets to the patient.

5. Yes，he can.

■ **Task 3**

1. penicillin   2. prescription   3. vitamin C effervescent tablets   4. directly   5. Excessive

■ **Task 4**

1. Rx   2. OTC   3. OTC   4. OCT   5. Rx

■ **Task 5**

Reference answer：

Relative of patient：Good afternoon.

Nurse：Good afternoon. What can I do for you，Sir?

Relative of patient：I want to consult something from you. My father is 80 years old. He has a cold. The doctor adviced me to give him some vitamin C. He always has the difficulty swallowing the tablets and he does not like the taste of chewable vitamin tablets.

Nurse: You can choose effervescent vitamin C as an alternative. In some instances, effervescent tablets can even be more affordable when compared to tablets and other forms.

Relative of patient: What is effervescent ?

Nurse: Effervescent tablets are tablets that are designed to break down rapidly when they are dropped into water or another liquid, releasing carbon dioxide in the process. The rapid breakdown causes the tablet to dissolve into a solution, and it often makes the solution frothy or fizzy.

Relative of patient: That means we can not eat effervescent tablets directly.

Nurse: Absolutely right.

Relative of patient: Can we add any liquids with it?

Nurse: The effervescent vitamin can be added to most liquids. It is recommended adding it to water to receive the maximum ascorbic acid benefit.

Relative of patient: Thanks so much.

Nurse: You are very welcome.

Activity 3　Introducing Community Health Service for the Elderly

■ **Task 1**

1. B　2. C　3. F　4. A　5. D　6. E　7. J　8. H　9. G　10. I

■ **Task 2**

1. needs; protection; improvement　2. spirit　3. public health practice　4. economic

■ **Task 3**

1. T　2. T　3. F　4. T　5. T

■ **Task 4**

1. community care

2. avoid illness

3. drug addiction; anxiety states

4. their quality of life; inappropriate reception

■ **Task 5**

Reference answer:

Nurse: Good morning.

Patient: Good morning.

Nurse: What can I help you, Sir?

Patient: My wife died two months ago. My son is too busy. I'm not in good health. I want to consult your community nursing home.

Nurse: Your choice is very correct. We are the best community nursing home in the city with professional medical staff and medical equipment. Could you tell me your medical history?

Patient: I have heart disease and high blood pressure. I take heart medicine regularly every day, but sometimes I forget it because I'm too old.

Nurse: If you come here, our nurse will remind you to take medicine. By the way, how old are you?

Patient: I'm 78.

Nurse：There are many old people of your age here. They live happily here.

Patient：Do you have any detailed information about your community nursing home? I want to take it back to my son and let him give me some suggestions.

Nurse：Of course. I will give some materials later. Meanwhile, I can show you around here and give you an introduction.

Patient：That would be great. Thank you.

Nurse：You are very welcome. This way, please.

Writing

Community Health Nursing

Community health services focus on health promotion, and disease prevention and management, which are designed to improve the health and wellbeing of local residents, as well as take pressure off the acute care health system.

Community health nurses work to improve the health and well – being of communities they serve by educating them about illness and disease prevention, safe health practices, nutrition, and wellness. They often provide treatment for poor, culturally diverse, and uninsured populations.

One of the primary functions of a community health nurse is to identify health problems in the community and to provide health care to patients who may not have access to, or be able to afford, medical services. They develop intervention plans to address the health, safety, and nutritional issues they discover and attempt to educate their patients about healthy choices that assist with disease and illness prevention.

Unit 9   Hospice Care

Warm – up Exercises

A – therapist   B – counselor   C – clergy   D – nurses   E – social workers   F – physicians

1. Therapists can assist the patient to maintain functional abilities for as long as possible; reduce the burden of care for the caregivers; assist in pain control.

2. Acounselor provids spiritual care for patients and their families. Through the establishment of ideas to ease the patient's fear and anxiety, so that they can feel at ease, and be full of hope.

3. Clergy can help the patients find relief in religious instruction, such as immortal, paradise. Listening is one of the greatest spiritual gifts clergy can give a suffering patient.

4. Hospice nurses manage pain and other symptoms, provide support to patients and families and assist in the process of death with dignity.

5. Social workers play an important role in planning and giving hospice care. They may be health professionals or lay people who provide services ranging from hands – on care to working in the hospice office or fundraising. Their support of family do not end with the death, but continute throughout the bereavement period.

6. The physician is in charge of the patient's care, write orders, see the patient for office visits, and complete and sign the death certificate.

Reading

■ **Task 1**

1. c   2. a   3. b   4. d   5. f   6. g   7. h   8. e   9. j   10. i

■ Task 2

1. comfort and dignity 2. patient's 3. on time 4. fatigue 5. Remaining stable

■ Task 3

1. Hospice care attends to the physical, emotional and sometimes spiritual needs of the terminally ill or elderly patients, focusing on palliation of their pain and symptoms, improving their quality of life and helping them die with more comfort and dignity.

2. Hospice care most often takes place in the patient's home or the home of a family member or friends. It also may be given in other locations, including nursing home, hospital or hospice center.

3. There are two principles for analgesic. One is Three – step Ladder Analgesic method proposed by WHO. The other is administer medication on time, not when necessary.

Listening and Speaking

Activity 1   Giving Bad News

■ Task 1

1. f 2. a 3. b 4. c 5. d 6. e

■ Task 2

1. N 2. U 3. R 4. S 5. E

■ Task 3

1. That is why

2. surgery; the symptom control

3. a course of chemotherapy

4. Your will to live

5. I will be with you

■ Task 4

1. (Naming) discouraged

2. (Respecting) impressed; appointments

3. (Respecting) amazing; inspiring

4. (Supporting) struggling with; control; as a team

Activity 2   Discussing Treatments

■ Task 1

1. C 2. B 3. A

■ Task 2

1. as 2. as possible 3. having a hard time 4. am tired of 5. make peace with God

6. take place 7. ensure

■ Task 3

1. e 2. a 3. d 4. b 5. c 6. f

■ Task 4

1. Hehas a high fever and slipped into a coma several times.

2. He had hoped the liver transplant would help him.

3. No, he doesn't. Because they all thought that this was his best chance for life. They don't want him to be taken away.

4. He said that he would never want to be kept alive by a machine.

5. He wants to be given a chance to have those last conversations, be comfortable at home, and be surrounded by family.

Activity 3　Supporting the Family of a Dying Patient

■ **Task 1**

1. a　2. c　3. b　4. e　5. d

■ **Task 2**

1. They sat around her and relived so many wonderful memories.

2. She was passionate about running, cycling, and yoga.

3. She's an awesome person.

■ **Task 3**

3　1　4　5　2　6

■ **Task 4**

1. passed on　2. are on their way; a couple of hours　3. delay moving　4. as much time as

5. be good for　6. clan customs　7. sense of humor.

Writing

There are five stages of grief. They are denial, anger, depression, bargaining, and acceptance.

Denial

"This can't be happening to me", No crying. Not accepting or even acknowledging the loss.

Anger

"Why me?", feelings of wanting to fight back.

Bargaining

Bargaining often takes place before the loss. Attempting to make deals with God to stop or change the loss. Begging, wishing, praying.

Depression

Overwhelming feelings of hopelessness, frustration, bitterness, self-pity, mourning loss of person as well as the hopes, dreams and plans for the future. Feeling lack of control, feeling numb. Perhaps feeling suicidal.

Acceptance

You have to accept the loss, not just try to bear it quietly. Realization that the person is gone (in death) that it is not their fault, they didn't leave you on purpose. Our goals turn toward personal growth. Stay with fond memories of person.

References

［1］李慧敏．护理英语会话［M］．北京：中国医药科技出版社，2013．

［2］朱彤．护士与新入院患者沟通技巧．中国民康医学．2013．

［3］方陵生，蒙蒙．CT 扫描与癌症风险［J］．中老年保健，2016（4 期）：50 – 51．

［4］赵玉沛，李宁，杨尹默，等．中国加速康复外科围术期管理专家共识（2016）［J］．中华外科杂志，54（6）：413 – 418，2016．

［5］手术室护理常用英语口语（2009）［J］．护理研究论丛，2009 年第 8 卷第 12 期（总第 91 期）．

［6］Virginia Allum，Patricia McGarr. Cambridge English For Nursing 1［M］．北京：中国青年出版社，2010．

［7］Virginia Allum, Patricia McGarr. Cambridge English For Nursing 2［M］．2 版．北京：中国青年出版社，2010．

［8］徐红莉，杨桂荣．涉外护理英语［M］．北京：对外经济贸易大学出版社，2013．

［9］Eric H. Glendinning, Ron Howard. Professional English in Use. 北京：人民邮电出版社，2013．

［10］雷子强．西方临床护理英语全攻略．北京：北京大学医学出版社，2007．